Herbs for Your Health

Steven Foster

Herbs for Your Health

A handy guide for knowing
and using 50 common herbs

Foreword by Mark Blumenthal

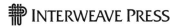 INTERWEAVE PRESS

Cover and interior design, Signorella Graphic Arts
Photography, Steven Foster and Thursday Plantation, Inc. (pages 94–95)
Production, Janice Paris

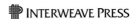 INTERWEAVE PRESS

Interweave Press, Inc.
201 East Fourth Street
Loveland, Colorado 80537-5655
USA

The information in this book should not be used as a substitute for advice from a qualified health-care practitioner. Dosage information is provided as a general guideline. Some medicinal herbs may cause allergic reactions in susceptible individuals, and others may not be right to use for particular health conditions.

Library of Congress Cataloging-in-Publication Data
Foster, Steven, 1957–
    Herbs for your health : a handy guide for knowing and using
50 common herbs / Steven Foster ; forward by Mark Blumenthal.
        p.   cm.
    Includes bibliographical references and index.
    ISBN   1-883010-27-6
    1. Herbs—Therapeutic use—Handbooks, manuals, etc.   2. Materia
medica, Vegetable—Handbooks, manuals, etc.   I. Title.
RM666.H33F674   1996
615' .321—dc20   96-30160
                                                       CIP

Printed in the United States of America
First Printing: 50M:996:QUE

Also by Steven Foster

A Field Guide to Medicinal Plants—Eastern and Central North America,
with James A. Duke

Echinacea—Nature's Immune Enhancer

Encyclopedia of Common Natural Ingredients Used in Food, Drugs, and Cosmetics,
with Albert Y. Leung

Forest Pharmacy—Medicinal Plants in American Forests

Herbal Bounty—The Gentle Art of Herb Culture

Herbal Emissaries—Bringing Chinese Herbs to the West, with Yue Chongxi

Herbal Renaissance—Growing, Using, and Understanding Herbs in the Modern World

Foreword

Herbs are hot! As the fastest-growing segment of the dietary supplement industry, herbs are no longer the domain of health-food stores, mail-order houses, and multilevel marketers. They are big business in places where big business is done—drugstores, supermarkets, and mass merchandisers. Herb sales in 1994 were 35 percent higher than 1993 sales in these outlets; total U. S. sales are expected to reach $2 billion in 1996.

The World Health Organization recognizes that herb use is increasing; it estimates that about 80 percent of the world's population still depends on traditional medicine for primary health care, and every form of traditional medicine uses herbs. In most countries, herbs are not "alternative" or "unconventional" but integral to the dominant health-care system. World herb sales were estimated at $12.4 billion in 1993, not counting Africa, South America, and parts of Asia (for which figures were not available). About half these sales were in western Europe and half again in Germany alone.

As the herb movement grows, products proliferate, and millions of Americans turn to them for health care and self-care. For those who may be exploring herbs for the first time, Steven Foster has written a book based on his respect for the traditions of the past and his knowledge of contemporary scientific research. He brings to this task a fervent love of plants, a thorough grasp of the botanical and clinical literature, and a selection of his exquisite herb photographs.

I first met Steven in 1978 at a "Boston Tea Party" staged in protest of the U. S. Food and Drug Administration ban on sassafras tea. The sassafras bark pitched over the sides of the Boston Tea Party Ship and Museum had been collected by Steven, then a young herbalist from Maine. We met again that year at the second annual Herb Trade Association Symposium on Herbs, a seminal event that brought backwoods herbalists, dropout herbalists, manufacturers of the budding herb industry, pharmacognosists, and ethnobotanists together for the first time. Almost twenty years have passed, the herb movement has blossomed and flourished, and Steven has emerged as one of the most knowledgeable and lucid writers in the field. He has published countless articles and numerous books, including the first on echinacea, which has established him as a leader among responsible echinacea promoters and educators.

In the sixteenth century, Paracelsus coined the term "essential oil" for the volatile oils that he believed represented the quintessence of many plants. Today, Steven Foster's writing and photography represent the quintessence of modern herbal literature.

—Mark Blumenthal
Founder and Executive Director
American Botanical Council
Editor, HerbalGram

To the teachers who profoundly impacted my life:

Sister Mildred Barker

Les Eastman

Dr. Shiu Ying Hu

Brother Theodore Johnson

Gail Scammon

Acknowledgments

This book could not have been published without the vision, assistance, and recommendations of many behind-the-scenes contributors. First, I thank Mark Blumenthal for his close review of the finished manuscript, for contributing the foreword, and for his wisdom and counsel during the last twenty years. Mary Pat Boian provided suggestions, research materials, and advice, and kept the office flowing when work on the book consumed me. Ellen Miller—thank you for your generous and invaluable help and support in pushing this project forward. A special thanks to Linda Ligon and Logan Chamberlain at Interweave Press for the vision. Bea Ferrigno provided the editorial prowess needed to meet a tight deadline and Betsy Strauch provided careful attention to detail. Thanks also to Kathleen Halloran and Jan Knight of Interweave who rearranged magazine deadlines to accommodate the flurry of work required for the book. I am grateful to Don Brown of Natural Products Research Consultants for providing some hard-to-find original research materials. Finally, thanks to my son Colin and daughter Abbey for dragging me out of the office when "You shouldn't be working."

—Steven Foster
Fayetteville, Arkansas
July 1996

Contents

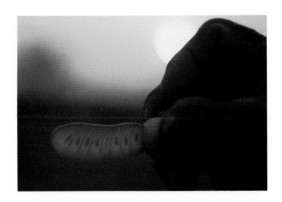

How To Use This Book

I live in a sea of herbal information, spending several thousand dollars a year on journals and books for my herb library and checking on-line services weekly for new information. When I was developing the plan for this book, the question uppermost in my mind was how to distill all this information into a digest of essential facts for the beginning herb user. I felt that it would be important for you to know what the plant is, where it comes from, and what it looks like. People interested in using herbs often want to know about traditional or historical use, so I include this information, as well as a summary of current research.

While the history of herbs is fascinating, I'm a skeptic at heart. Tell me an herb is good for this or that, or will enhance my health in a certain manner, and I will say "Prove it." In following up traditional claims for herbs, I have examined the scientific literature for laboratory or human studies that back or refute those claims. References to the original studies begin on page 105.

Once you have an herb, you want to know how to prepare and use it. You want to know the appropriate dose. The dosage information in this book draws heavily on monographs published by Germany's Commission E, a special governmental advisory group that establishes regulatory guidelines for herbal medicines in that country. These regulations include what benefits the herb can be expected to produce, the dose, side effects, warnings, contraindications, and interactions with other substances. The American Botanical Council, a nonprofit organization in Austin, Texas that publishes the magazine *HerbalGram*, will soon publish English translations of the German Commission E regulations on herbs. Those translations provide the basis for guidelines on dosage and cautions in this book. Please remember this: **any substance—whether derived from natural or man-made sources—may produce adverse reactions in some people.** Always make sure to heed cautions about herbs and share them with your health-care practitioner. This procedure is part of using herbs responsibly.

This book is designed as a quick reference guide to the fifty most commonly used herbs available in the United States as dietary supplements. The profile of each herb includes:

- common and botanical name(s)

- a brief history of its traditional uses

- a summary of the credible scientific reports, which may validate or challenge traditional claims for the herb's efficacy

- brief descriptions of conditions and symptoms for which the herb
- has clinically demonstrated effects and descriptions of its action(s)

- forms in which it is available in the United States

- a guide to proper dosage

- cautions or contraindications.

Guidelines for Selecting Herbs

Health or natural-food stores, even pharmacies, offer a bewildering array of herb products—dozens of brightly colored packages, all screaming "Buy me!" Confronted by herbs in bulk, capsules, tablets, tinctures, and many other product forms, you stand there and scratch your head. You hesitate to ask the clerk what might be a stupid question. Then again, the clerk may not know enough to be helpful. Don't be afraid to ask questions, though, or insist on validation of any claims made. If a claim sounds too good to be true, it probably is.

When I am looking for a particular herb, several factors determine the form I select. If I am going to make my own preparation, or an herbal tea, I usually select bulk herbs. Teas formulated for specific purposes, such as relaxation at bedtime, are quite convenient. When I need an herb for a particular application, I choose products standardized to contain a certain amount of active constituents, often from European phytomedicine firms whose products are backed by good studies on their use and safety. These are more expensive than bulk herbs, but in this case you do get what you pay for.

In this book's herb profiles, you will find information similar to what you might see on the label of a standardized product. If you are looking for a St.-John's-wort preparation, for example, you can scan the shelves and find many choices. A simple package may exclaim "St.-John's-wort" on its label, but if the side panel doesn't mention anything about the herb contained inside, or if the plant's name is misspelled, it gives me little confidence that the company knows what it's doing. If, however, the label on another package specifies a daily dose, tells me the product is standardized to contain 0.2% percent hypericin, and warns me not to take it before going out in the sun, then I have enough information to make a decision. I will buy the second product, even though it costs twice as much as the first. When shopping for a product that will give me ginseng's subtle long-term tonic effects, I'll choose a standardized Asian ginseng extract, either in liquid or capsule form, over a cheaper product that lists ginseng after fructose in the ingredients. If I simply want something to calm my digestive system or quiet my overactive mind before bed, a pleasant cup of peppermint or chamomile tea is all I wish.

In these ways, this book should help you become a more savvy buyer and user of herb products.

Guidelines for Preparing and Using Herbs

Dosage is often best left to health-care practitioners to determine for their patients. In the case of manufactured products, follow label instructions. Much of the dosage information in this book is drawn from Germany's Commission E monographs, the Chinese pharmacopoeia, or other authoritative works. Because the U. S. system of measurement is much less precise in small measures than the metric system, the weights of herbs in this book are expressed in grams. Nevertheless, you can roughly translate metric measurements into U. S. measurements.

Dry measurements:

  5 g = 1 teaspoonful of dried powdered herb
  10 g = 2 teaspoonfuls of dried powdered herb
  15 g = 1 tablespoonful (or about ½ ounce) of dried powdered herb

Fluid measures of herbs are usually expressed in milliliters. One milliliter is one-thousandth of a liter or about one-thirtieth of a fluid ounce. There are about two tablespoons (6 teaspoons) in an ounce. Herbal doses in milliliters may be translated to doses in drops or teaspoons. In liquid measure, a teaspoon contains 5 ml or roughly 50 drops; ¼ teaspoon contains 1 ml or about 10 drops.

To make life simpler, I often advise you to follow the manufacturer's recommended dosages for capsules, tablets, tinctures, and especially products standardized to deliver a certain weight of an extract or chemical component. (Capsules and tablets generally contain only the powdered herb.)

A tea or infusion is the simplest way to prepare herbs. A single dose generally consists of a quantity of a given herb steeped in a cup of water. Simply bring water to the boil, pour it over the herb in a teapot or cup, cover, steep for at least fifteen minutes, and then drink the liquid.

A decoction, often used for roots and barks, is somewhat akin to a "soup" of the herb. Bring a quart of water to the boil, add the appropriate amount of herb, then simmer for 30–60 minutes, or until one-half to two-thirds of the original volume of liquid has been evaporated or absorbed by the herb. Then strain out the herb and drink about half a cup of the liquid two to three times a day.

A tincture is made by soaking an herb in a solution of ethyl alcohol or by percolating alcohol through it. A product label may carry a ratio such as 5:1. This means that there are five parts of herb by liquid unit of measure to one part of alcohol. A 5:1 tincture is five times as strong as a 1:1 tincture.

An extract is an herb product made by treating an herb with a solvent such as water, alcohol, or hexane. The solution containing the soluble part of the herb is separated from the insoluble part. The solvent itself, in the case of hexane, for example, may also be removed. Extraction can be a very complex process involving a dozen or more steps, or a relatively simple matter. (A tincture is a simple extract.) Extracts are more concentrated than crude dried herbs. Both liquid and dry extracts are available.

Essential, or volatile, oils are the hallmark of aromatic herbs. With a 10× hand lens, look closely at the underside of a mint leaf. You will see little liquid beads. These are the essential oil glands. Plants produce essential oils to protect themselves from insects or other invaders, or to attract pollinators. The oils also contain the chemicals responsible for the plant's flavor, fragrance, and often its medicinal value. Essential oils are produced commercially, most often by steam distillation. The fresh or dried herb is heated in a big tub of water and the resulting steam passes through a condenser, which cools it. The liquid is then collected in a container. Because the water and essential oil are of different densities, one floats on top of the other, and the essential oil can be drawn off the top or bottom of the container. Essential oils are highly concentrated: an acre of peppermint may produce a ton of dried leaf but only 12 pounds of peppermint oil. Essential oils evaporate readily. They should be used in minute amounts and with appropriate cautions. They can be highly irritating if ingested or if they contact the skin or mucous membranes. Fixed oils, such as almond oil or olive oil, by contrast contain fatty substances and do not evaporate, nor are they soluble in water.

Introduction

Herbs have been the main source of medicine throughout human history. That they are still widely used today is not a throwback to the Dark Ages but an indication that herbs are a growing part of modern, high-tech medicine: about 25 percent of today's prescription drugs contain chemicals derived from plants. Some 119 chemical substances from 91 plants are now used in Western medicine. Of these, 74 percent were folk medicines brought to our pharmacies through scientific research. Researchers today examine folk or historical uses of plants to find new drugs for cancer, AIDS, and even the common cold.

In Western countries, contemporary herbal medicine is based on European phytomedicine. Derived from plants or plant parts, phytomedicines are not isolated chemicals but preparations from an entire plant or from its root, leaf, flower, or fruit. Thus, such well-known compounds as menthol (from peppermint), or digitoxin (from foxglove) are not considered phytomedicines. The European phytomedicine market is estimated at more than $8 billion in annual sales, 70 percent of which are made in Germany, a country with a rich tradition of herbal medicine. One survey revealed that 76 percent of German women drink herbal teas for health benefits, and more than 50 percent take herbal remedies in the early stages of illness. Germany also has a favorable regulatory system that permits well-researched, well-documented herbs to be sold as drugs. Herbs widely used in Europe for many years are now becoming popular in the United States as dietary supplements.

Many Americans are now taking greater responsibility for their own health and are consequently seeking alternatives to conventional medicine such as prevention through attention to diet, exercise, and the use of dietary supplements and herbs. Millions of consumers, frustrated with the cost of medical care and the not-so-wonderful side effects of wonder drugs, are turning to these health-care alternatives. According to the *New England Journal of Medicine*, Americans spent $13.7 billion on alternative forms of health care in 1990. As we move into the twenty-first century, herbs will no doubt be increasingly important in the maintenance of health and in the prevention and treatment of disease.

In the United States, herb products are regulated as foods rather than drugs, unless a product has been approved as a nonprescription (over-the-counter) or prescription drug. Most herb products are now designated as dietary supplements. The Dietary Supplement Health and Education Act of 1994 (DSHEA, popularly pronounced D-shay) laid the foundation for federal regulation of dietary supplements, including herbs. DSHEA seeks to guarantee availability of products; allow truthful, non-misleading scientific information to be used in conjunction with their sale; and give consumers some information on the product's benefits, as well as appropriate cautions. While DSHEA preserves existing safety standards in the Food, Drug and Cosmetic Act, it offers additional safeguards to protect consumers from unreasonable risk or injury. The bill also places the burden of proof that a dietary supplement is adulterated or unsafe on the government, which must now present its evidence that a dietary supplement is unsafe in court. Formerly, the U. S. Food and Drug Administration (FDA) could simply order a manufacturer to stop selling a questionable product.

DSHEA also permits third-party information such as publications, articles, chapters in books, and scientific reports to support the sale of dietary supplements. The information must not be false or misleading, nor may it promote a particular manufacturer or product brand; it must present a balanced view of the scientific information and, if displayed in a store, must be physically separate from the product and free of any appendages such as stickers.

The bill allows product labels to describe effects on general well-being or on structure or function in humans, but drug claims may not be made. For example, a manufacturer may claim that a garlic product helps to reduce cholesterol—but not that *garlic* helps to reduce cholesterol, thereby reducing the risk of heart disease. Dietary supplement labels with structure or function claims must also carry a disclaimer: *This statement has not been evaluated by the Food and Drug*

Administration. This product is not intended to diagnose, treat, cure, or prevent any disease. When this disclaimer appears on a product label or in advertising, a structure or function claim is being made, and presumably, the manufacturer can substantiate it. The manufacturer must also notify the Secretary of Health and Human Services within thirty days of making such a claim.

DSHEA has also established an Office of Dietary Supplements within the National Institutes of Health to conduct, coordinate, and collect data on dietary supplements and to advise the Secretary of Health and Human Services. A separate Presidential Dietary Supplement Commission has been formed to study and make recommendations on dietary supplement labels and is to issue a report of its findings.

Profiles of Herbs

Alfalfa

Medicago sativa

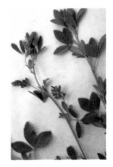

Source: Alfalfa is the dried leaf of a well-known pea family member, with purple flowers and clover-like leaves. It is native to western Asia and the eastern Mediterranean region and is widely grown as fodder for farm animals.

Traditional Use: Alfalfa leaf has been used in tea and dietary supplements to help increase appetite and vitality, reduce water retention, and as a stimulant for digestion and bowel action. It is a folk treatment for rheumatoid arthritis, diabetes, and preventing absorption of cholesterol from the diet. Its use for loss of energy due to indigestion, dyspepsia, anemia, loss of appetite, and poor assimilation began in the early 1900s with American physicians who specialized in herbal medicine. Dr. Ben A. Bradley of Hamlet, Ohio, wrote in 1915: "I find in Alfalfa, after about seven years' clinical tests in my practice and on myself, a superlative restorative tonic. . . . It rejuvenates the whole system by increasing the strength, vim, vigor, and vitality of the patient."

Current Status: Alfalfa has been thoroughly studied as an animal feed but not as an herbal medicine for humans. Animal studies suggest it can prevent high cholesterol in animals on high-fat diets. Compounds in the plant may decrease intestinal absorption of cholesterol and reduce atherosclerotic plaque.

Alfalfa is high in protein and contains vitamins A, B_1, B_6, B_{12}, C, E, and K_1, along with the minerals calcium, potassium, phosphorus, iron, and zinc.

Despite its widespread use as a dietary supplement, there are no human studies of its claimed benefits. Alfalfa would be a good subject for further research.

Product forms: Alfalfa is available as dried leaf, tablets, capsules, extracts, health drinks, tea, and in other forms.

Dosage: One or two 500-mg capsules or tablets a day. No therapeutic dosage has been established.

Cautions: Moderate use of alfalfa products is not associated with side effects. A case of allergic reaction (from contamination with grass pollen) in alfalfa tablets has been reported. Eating alfalfa seeds or sprouts has been linked to systemic lupus erythematosus (SLE), a condition characterized by inflammation of connective tissue. In two instances, alfalfa sprouts caused the recurrence of SLE in individuals who had been treated for the condition. Those diagnosed with SLE should avoid alfalfa products. Consuming large quantities of the seeds has also produced reversible blood abnormalities. The compound responsible for ill effects is canavanine.

Actions

Appetite stimulant

Nutritive

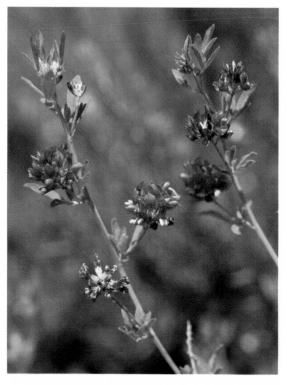

Aloe

Aloe vera (formerly *A. barbadensis*)

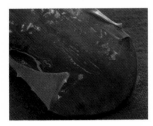

Source: If any herb claims to be America's number one folk remedy, it is aloe. Aloe is a succulent perennial of the lily family native to Africa and commercially grown in southern Texas and Mexico. The leaf contains a gooey gel; the outer leaf tissue produces a bitter yellow juice, known as drug aloe, once a widely used laxative. Aloe gel should not be confused with drug aloe.

Traditional Use: Aloe gel has been used to treat inflammation for more than 2,500 years. The fresh gel is widely used as a folk medicine for minor burns and sunburn, as well as minor cuts and scrapes. Aloe gel is also used in beverages commonly sold as "aloe juice". Aloe gel, mixed with water, citric acid, fruit juices, and preservatives is also marketed as "aloe juice", touted as a digestive aid or folk remedy for arthritis, stomach ulcers, diabetes, and other conditions.

Current Status: Modern clinical use of aloe gel began in the 1930s, but favorable case histories did not provide conclusive evidence of its effectiveness. Recent studies have documented that aloe gel promotes wound healing and is of therapeutic value in thermal injuries and a variety of soft-tissue injuries. In animal studies, it prevented progressive skin damage that usually follows burns, frostbite, and electrical injuries. Aloe gel penetrates injured tissue, relieves pain and inflammation, and dilates capillaries, increasing blood supply to the injury. Ultimately, aloe gel increases both tensile strength at the wound site and healing activity in the space between cells, thus helping to promote recovery.

Several animal studies failed to demonstrate aloe's anti-ulcer or antidiabetic potential, thus refuting some of its traditional uses. Studies of purified compounds from a Japanese species, *A. arborescens* (Kidachi aloe), however, did show an antidiabetic effect, as well as inhibition of stomach secretions and lesions. More research is needed.

Preparations: Aloe gel can be obtained from the living plant. It is an ingredient in many sunscreens, skin creams, lotions, and other cosmetics. Some products boast of aloe content but contain too little to do any good. Aloe juice comes in various concentrations; highly concentrated products degrade readily. Read the product label for information on addition of carriers such as gums, sugars, or starches.

Dosage: Fresh aloe gel can be obtained by cutting a leaf lengthwise and scraping the gel out with a spoon. It can also be obtained by cutting a leaf from the base of the plant and squeezing it. Apply externally as needed; discontinue if burning or irritation occurs. For commercial aloe juice, 1 tsp after meals is often suggested. Read the product label for specific recommendations.

Cautions: The topical use of aloe gel or aloe gel products does not usually produce adverse reactions or side effects. However, there are reports of skin burning following dermal abrasion for removal of acne scars. Rare instances of contact dermatitis (rash) have also been reported. Taking more than the recommended dose of aloe juice may produce a laxative effect. You can get too much of a good thing.

Symptoms

First-degree burns

Cuts and abrasions

Actions

Promotes wound healing

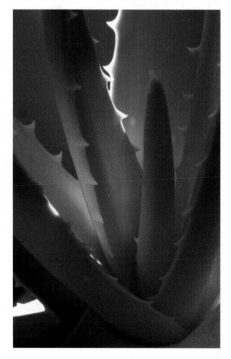

Astragalus

Astragalus membranaceus

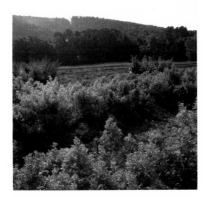

Sources: Astragalus is the root of *A. membranaceus* or *A. membranaceus* var. *mongholicus (A. mongholicus),* members of the pea family native to northeast China, where astralagus is commercially grown. Cultivation has also begun in the United States. In China, the root is called *huang-qi.*

Traditional Use: Astragalus is first mentioned in the 2,000-year-old classic, *Shen Nong Ben Cao Jing.*
The Chinese name huang-qi means "yellow leader" because it is one of the superior tonic roots in traditional Chinese medicine. It has been used to invigorate vital energy (qi) and in prescriptions for shortness of breath, general weakness, and lack of appetite; also as a diuretic, and for the treatment of colds, flu, stomach ulcers, and diabetes. It is widely used in modern herbal practice in China.

Current Status: As one of the important tonic herbs in Chinese medicine, astragalus has been extensively studied by Asian scientists. Numerous studies confirm its immunostimulant, antibacterial, antiviral, anti-inflammatory, adaptogenic, and diuretic effects. It also improves stamina. No single compound is responsible for its wide-ranging effects, though polysaccharides are involved in immunostimulant activity.

Since 1975, astragalus has been used in China in cancer patients undergoing radiation treatment and chemotherapy. Conventional cancer treatments reduce the function of the immune system, so astragalus helps return it to normal function. Its positive effects on the cardiovascular system have also been extensively studied in China.

In the early 1980s, researchers in Houston, Texas, studied the effects of astragalus on nineteen cancer patients and fifteen healthy individuals. A chemical fraction extract of astragalus was found to restore T-cell function in 90 percent of the cancer patients to levels observed in the healthy subjects. The studies showed that astragalus had a strong immunostimulant effect, thus establishing a basis for using it to improve response in cancer patients. Chinese studies show that immunostimulant effects include enhancing the particle ingestion capacity of white blood cells.

Preparations: The dried sliced root, which looks like a tongue depressor, is the usual form of the crude herb supplied from Chinese sources. Tinctures, tablets, capsules, powdered herb, extracts, and combination products are found in the American herb market. It is often combined with ginseng.

Dosage: In Chinese tradition, 9–15 g of the dried sliced herb are made into a thick tea by simmering for several hours. Typically, American capsules deliver a dose of about 0.5 g. Two average capsules three times a day would be equivalent to a dose of 3 g.

Cautions: No side effects or adverse reactions have been reported.

Symptons

Colds

Flu

Infections, minor

Actions

Adaptogen (tonic)

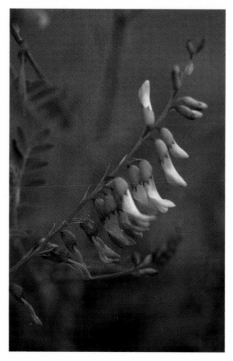

Bearberry

Arctostaphylos uva-ursi

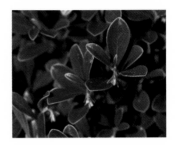

Source: Bearberry, or uva-ursi, is the leaf of a member of the heath family. This trailing, low-growing evergreen shrub is found in cool temperate regions of the Northern Hemisphere, including North America, Europe, and Asia. Most of the leaf in commerce is wild-harvested.

Traditional Use: Traditionally, the astringent leaves have been used for diarrhea and dysentery and for bladder infections and other afflictions of the urinary tract. It has also been a folk medicine in the treatment of bronchitis. Bearberry was long used as a urinary antiseptic by physicians; it was official in the *U. S. Pharmacopoeia* from 1820 to 1926.

Current Status: Bearberry is an excellent example of an herb whose safe and effective use is far more complicated than simply preparing an herb tea. While often described as a "diuretic", bearberry does not strongly promote urination but rather serves as a urinary antiseptic. It contains arbutin and methylarbutin which are transformed into hydroquinone in the intestine. After this compound has been absorbed by the intestine, it binds to other compounds in the urine (*if* the urine is alkaline), forming two additional chemicals which kill or inhibit bacteria in the urinary tract. In Germany, bearberry is approved as a urinary antiseptic.

Preparations: Bearberry is formulated in capsules, tablets, tea, and tinctures. The dried herb is generally used. In Europe, coated tablets, which dissolve in the intestinal tract instead of the stomach, are available, minimizing potential side effects (see below). The leaves should contain at least 6 percent arbutin for reliable effects.

Dosage: Traditionally, about 10 g (⅓ ounce) of dried leaves are soaked in a quart of cold water for 24 hours; then the leaves are removed, and the cold infusion is simmered down to half a quart. The cold water soak reduces the amount of tannins, which can irritate the stomach. The decoction is taken in 1–2 fl oz doses three times a day. In order for it to be effective, the urine must be alka-

Bearberry

line—a couple of teaspoons of sodium bicarbonate (baking soda) in a glass of water each day will help to accomplish this.

Cautions: Bearberry is high in tannins, which can produce stomachache, nausea, and vomiting. If you have a weak stomach, avoid bearberry. It is generally not recommended for children. Use should not be continued for more than a week except under the direction of a physician, as overuse may cause liver damage. It should not be used for suspected kidney disorders, as kidney disease cannot be self-diagnosed. Avoid during pregnancy.

Symptoms

Urinary tract infections, mild

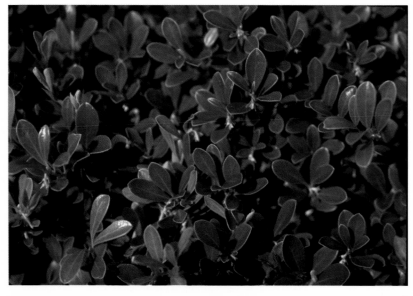

Bilberry

Vaccinium myrtillus

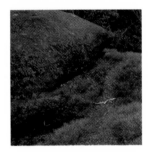

Source: Bilberry, a relative of blueberry, belongs to the heath family. A small shrub with sweet black berries, it grows in heaths and woods of northern Europe, as well as western Asia, and the Rocky Mountains of western North America. The berries and leaves are used.

Traditional Use: An ancient food plant of Europe, bilberry emerged as a medicinal herb in the sixteenth century. The leaves were used for their astringent, tonic, anti-inflammatory, and antiseptic qualities.

The dried berry tea was used as an astringent for diarrhea and dysentery, a diuretic, and a cooling nutritive tonic; also to prevent scurvy (vitamin C deficiency) and to stop bleeding. It is also used as an astringent and disinfectant for mouth inflammations.

During the Second World War, pilots in the British Royal Air Force reported improved night vision after eating bilberry jam. In the 1960s, these reports led Italian and French scientists to research the berries for their effects on vision problems.

Current Status: In Europe, herbal preparations of bilberry fruit are used to enhance poor microcirculation, thus improving eye conditions such as night blindness and diabetic retinopathy. Pigments called anthocyanosides help regenerate a pigment in the retina which is essential for the eye to adapt to light.

Fragility of capillaries is a common condition in the elderly which can result in a tendency to bruise easily. Weak capillaries are associated with poor blood circulation to connective tissues and with inflammatory conditions such as arthritis. Anthocyanosides in bilberry strengthen capillaries by protecting them from free radical damage. They also stimulate the formation of healthy connective tissue and aid in the formation of new capillaries. Bilberry may reduce blood platelet stickiness (platelet aggregation), a risk factor associated with atherosclerosis. Bilberry is recommended for managing varicose veins and hemorrhoids, and rebuilding healthy connective tissue, but unfortunately most studies have involved animals or only a small number of humans. In Germany, the dried berries are sold for the traditional use of treating mild diarrhea and minor inflammations of the mucous membranes of the throat and mouth. More studies are needed.

Preparations: Tablets and capsules of the dried fruits are available, as well as products standardized to 25 percent anthocyanosides. Standardized products may be expected to produce more predictable results.

Dosage: The dried ripe berries are used in a dose of 20 to 60 g daily, prepared as a tea. Standardized products are taken at a dose of 240 to 480 mg per day, divided into two or three doses.

Cautions: No side effects, contraindications, or interactions with other drugs have been reported.

Symptoms

Atherosclerosis

Diarrhea

Hemorrhoids

Mouth and throat inflammation

Tendency to bruising

Varicose veins

Actions

Improves microcirculation

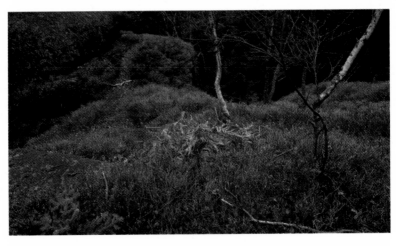

Black cohosh

Cimicifuga racemosa

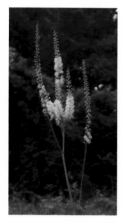

Source: Black cohosh, the root of a member of the buttercup family, is found in rich woods of the eastern deciduous forest from southern Ontario south to Georgia, west to Arkansas, and north to Wisconsin. Most of the root is wild-harvested, while some is grown commercially in Europe.

Traditional Use: Among Native Americans and early settlers in North America, black cohosh root was an important folk medicine for menstrual irregularities and as an aid in childbirth. Adopted in medical practice in the early nineteenth century, it had a great reputation as an anti-inflammatory for arthritis and rheumatism; for normalizing suppressed or painful menses; and for relieving pain after childbirth. It was also used for nervous disorders. The root was an official drug in the *U. S. Pharmacopoeia* from 1820 to 1926.

Current Status: Black cohosh is approved for use in Germany for the treatment of premenstrual symptoms, painful or difficult menstruation, and for menopausal symptoms such as hot flashes. A number of studies have confirmed its mild sedative and anti-inflammatory activity. An isoflavone in the root binds to estrogen receptors, producing estrogenlike activity. As ovarian function declines during menopause, estrogen production also declines and luteinizing-hormone (LH) increases. These changes are associated with hot flashes. In one study an alcohol extract of black cohosh lowered LH in both animals and women, reducing hot flashes. Three as yet unidentified compounds are believed to work in concert to produce the benefits (Duker).

Another study compared the effects of conventional estrogen replacement therapy with black cohosh in sixty women less than forty years old who had complete hysterectomies and were experiencing menopauselike symptoms. In all groups, a reduction in LH was observed. Black cohosh treatment was comparable to conventional treatment. Despite these successes and the long tradition of use, more clinical research is necessary.

Preparations: In the American market, tablets, capsules and tinctures are generally available, as well as the dried root.

Dosage: A decoction of 0.3 to 2 g (up to ½ tsp) of the dried cut-and-sifted root is used. In Germany the daily dose is an extract with 40 mg of the herb in 40–60 percent alcohol. Use is limited to six months. Follow label instructions for commercial products.

Cautions: No contraindications or drug interactions are reported, though some women have experienced upset stomach from use of black cohosh preparations. No long-term toxicity studies have been conducted.

Symptoms

Menopausal difficulties

Menstrual difficulties

PMS

Actions

Anti-inflammatory

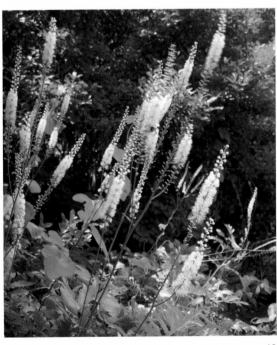

Calendula

Calendula officinalis

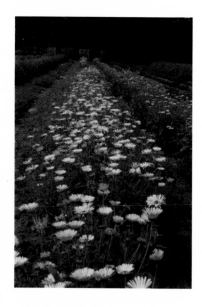

Source: Also known as pot marigold (not to be confused with common garden marigolds, *Tagetes* species), calendula is the dried flower of a member of the aster family native to south-central Europe and northern Africa. It is an annual commonly grown in gardens for its bright display of yellow or orange flowers.

Traditional Use: The flowers have been applied to cuts and wounds, burns and bruises, and used as a tea for gastric ulcers and other stomach ailments, for jaundice and other conditions.

Current Status: Calendula preparations are approved in Germany and other European countries for topical use on slow-to-heal wounds and for ulcerations on the leg. A gargle or tea is also used to reduce inflammation of the mouth or sore throat. Most human studies of the plant have been conducted in eastern European countries and involve only small numbers of patients. They indicate that extracts of the herb may be of use in treating duodenal ulcers and may help surgical wounds heal more rapidly.

Pharmacological studies, most involving animals, have confirmed a wide range of activities. Calendula extracts are anti-inflammatory, antiviral, and stimulate the immune system to increase the particle ingestion capacity of white blood cells. (In this respect, calendula is similar to echinacea.) Triterpenoids in calendula have recently been linked to its anti-inflammatory activity. In addition, calendula increases granulation at the site of a wound, promoting metabolism of proteins and collagen—in other words, helping grow new healthy cells. Topical calendula preparations are widely accepted in Europe for treating inflammation of the skin and mucous membranes, slow-to-heal wounds, mild burns, and sunburn.

14

Preparations: The dried flower, salves, and tinctures are available.

Dosage: Internally, a tea of 1–5 g of the herb in a cup of water is taken three times a day. For tinctures, 5 to 40 drops are taken three times a day. Externally, the tincture is dabbed on with cotton; a fresh poultice may be used, or salves, following label directions.

Cautions: Generally no side effects or contraindications have been reported. Persons allergic to pollen of other members of the aster family, such as ragweed, may also be allergic to calendula. One case of a severe allergic reaction to the tea was reported in Russia.

Symptoms

First-degree burns

Mouth and throat infections

Sore throat

Actions

Promotes wound healing

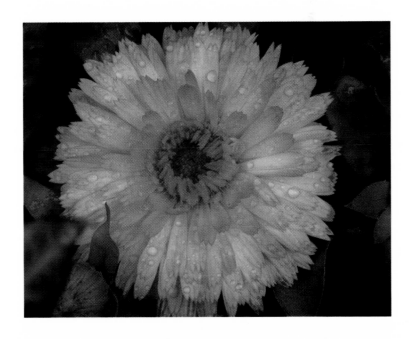

Cascara sagrada

Rhamnus purshiana

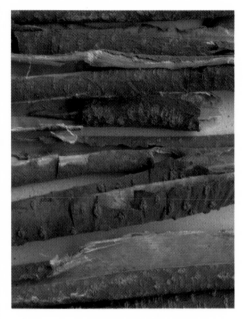

Source: Cascara sagrada is the dried, aged bark of a small tree in the buckthorn family native to the Pacific Northwest. The bark is harvested mostly from wild trees in Oregon, Washington, and southern British Columbia. The bark is aged for a year so that the active principles become milder, as freshly dried bark produces too strong a laxative for safe use; it also contains a compound that induces vomiting.

Traditional Use: The name cascara sagrada is Spanish for "sacred bark". Long used as a laxative by Native American groups of the northwest Pacific coast, cascara sagrada bark was not introduced into formal medical practice in the United States until 1877. In 1890, it replaced the berries of the European buckthorn (*R. catharticus*) as an official laxative. It is still used in over-the-counter laxatives available in every pharmacy in the United States.

Current Status: Dried, aged cascara sagrada bark is widely accepted as a mild and effective treatment for chronic constipation. The bark contains compounds called anthraquinones (cascarosides A and B) which are transformed by intestinal bacteria into substances that increase peristalsis in the large intestine and help restore its tone.

Preparations: Cascara sagrada is available in capsules, extracts, and as dried bark. It is a little silly, however, to make a tea of the extremely bitter bark when you can go to a pharmacy for a fluid extract, or to a health food store for capsules, both of which are much easier to take.

Dosage: The usual dose is 1 ml (about 10 drops) of the fluid extract. *Follow label instructions.*

Cautions: Only the aged bark should be used. If you have chronic constipation, see your doctor for other approaches to avoid laxative dependency.

Symptoms

Constipation

Actions

Laxative

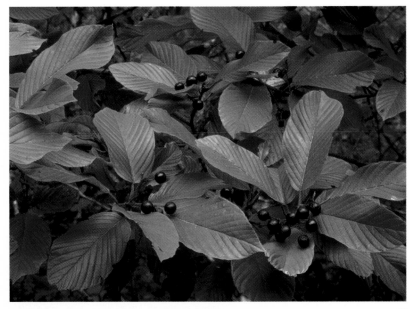

Cat's-claw

Uncaria tomentosa, U. guianensis

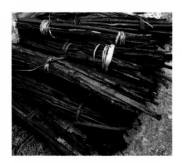

Sources: Cat's-claw (uña de gato) comes from the stem and root of two Amazonian woody vines belonging to the madder family. Both species are used interchangeably in South America. Commercial supplies are wild-harvested in Peru and Brazil.

Traditional Use: The Piura Indians used a bark decoction of *U. guianensis* to treat inflammation, rheumatism, gastric ulcers and tumors, and as a contraceptive. Indian groups in Colombia and Guyana use it for dysentery. *U. tomentosa* is a South American folk medicine for intestinal ailments, gastric ulcers, arthritis, wounds, and cancer. Popular use in North America started in the 1990s.

Current Status: Reports of successful use as a South American folk remedy for cancer prompted scientists in Germany, Austria, and Italy to take a closer look at cat's-claw. Compounds called proanthocyanidins were found to inhibit tumor growth in animals in the 1970s. Studies at the University of Munich in 1985 found several alkaloids in *U. tomentosa* root with significant immunostimulant activity. In 1993 Italian researchers found new compounds, quinovic glycosides, which showed antiviral, antimutagenic, and antioxidant effects in preliminary pharmacological tests. An Austrian research group found several alkaloids, including uncarine F, inhibit the growth of tumor cells in laboratory tests. Root material may be as much as four times stronger than stem bark.

In Germany and Austria, standardized cat's-claw extracts have been given to cancer patients under a physician's care to stimulate their immune system. They have also been used in cases of rheumatoid arthritis, allergies, herpes infections, gastric ulcers, gastritis, and AIDS. The products are registered pharmaceuticals in these countries and are available only by prescription. Controlled clinical studies are underway, but results to date are inconclusive.

Preparations: The dried cut-and-sifted root and stem, powdered root and stem, capsules, tinctures, tablets, and extracts standardized for total alkaloid content are now available in the American market.

Dosage: A dose of 20–60 mg per day of a standardized dry extract is used by German and Austrian physicians. A decoction is made by simmering 20 g (about 1 tbsp) of pulverized root in a liter of water at 176°F for 45 minutes. The adult dose is 60 ml (1 tsp) of the decoction added to 60 ml of hot water before breakfast.

Cautions: Like other immunostimulants, cat's-claw should be avoided in diseases of the immune system itself, such as tuberculosis, multiple sclerosis, and HIV infection. [It is not known to be safe for children or pregnant or nursing women.] In Germany and Austria, standardized products are not allowed to be combined with therapies involving hormones, insulin, fresh blood plasma, vaccines, or in certain other special situations. Consult a physician before using cat's-claw.

Actions

Anti-inflammatory

Immunostimulant

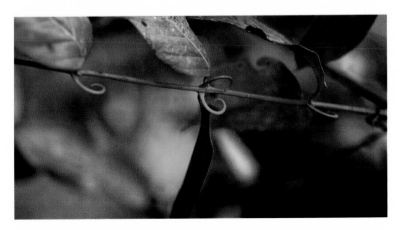

Cayenne

Capsicum annuum, C. frutescens

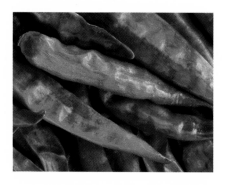

Source: Cayenne is the pungent dried fruit of a highly variable species in the nightshade family that also gives us paprika, bell peppers, and jalapeños. [*C. frutescens* also produces hot peppers that are used medicinally.] Cayenne originates in the tropical Americas and is grown worldwide.

Traditional Use: The ancient Maya used cayenne to treat mouth sores and inflamed gums. Herbal use as a stimulant began with Samuel Thomson (1769–1843), who used it to "produce a strong heat in the body" and "restore digestive powers". In the 1970s John Christopher promoted cayenne as a circulatory stimulant, claiming that "it feeds the necessary elements into the cell structure of the arteries, veins and capillaries so that these regain the elasticity of youth again, and the blood pressure adjusts itself to normal."

Current Status: The popular belief that cayenne stimulates digestion and circulation has no scientific proof; in Germany, therefore, cayenne products are not permitted to carry claims about stimulating digestion or circulation. It does, however, contain carotenoids and vitamins C and E; these antioxidants protect against free radicals, oxygen compounds that can damage cell membranes and disturb metabolic pathways. Consumption of carotenoids is associated with a reduced risk of cancer and enhances the activity of various immune-system cells. The carotenoids in red peppers have been shown clinically to improve lifespan in primates.

Capsaicin, the source of cayenne's bite, is used in minute amounts in topical pharmaceutical products to treat pain at the site of an apparently healed infection, rheumatoid and osteoarthritis, and shingles. (The whole herb itself is not used in this way.)

Preparations: Cayenne is available fresh or as whole dried fruit, dried powdered fruit, and in capsules, tablets, and tinctures. Both over-the-counter and prescription ointments and creams containing

Cayenne

capsaicin are prescribed by physicians. The concentration of capsaicin in topical preparations is typically 0.025 to 0.075 percent. Topical products should be used under a physician's direction.

Dosage: Use freely as a spice. A tea can be made with $\frac{1}{2}$ to 1 tsp of the powdered fruit in a cup of water. Good luck!

Cautions: Cayenne's pungent principle, capsaicin, is a highly toxic irritant in its pure form. Capsaicin is not water soluble, so it is difficult to wash it off one's hands after handling hot peppers. Scientists working with capsaicin protect themselves with space suit-like garb. Handling hot peppers can cause burning skin irritation, a condition called "Hunan hand" from the spicy cuisine of Hunan, China.

Actions

Antioxidant

Nutritive

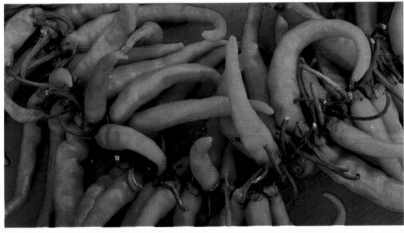

Chamomile

Matricaria recutita (formerly M. chamomilla, Chamomilla recutita)

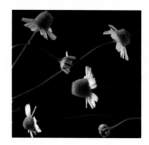

Source: Chamomile (or German camomile) is the dried flower head of an annual member of the aster family. The primary chamomile of commerce, it is grown in Hungary, the Czech Republic, Slovakia, Germany, Argentina, and Egypt. Roman (or English) chamomile, the flower of the perennial *Chamaemelum nobile* (formerly *Anthemis nobilis*), is less frequently seen in the American market.

Traditional Use: According to Varro Tyler, Germans call chamomile *alles zutraut*—"capable of anything". A Slovakian chamomile specialist, Ivan Salamon, states:

> Chamomile is the most favored and most used medicinal plant in Slovakia. Our folk saying indicates that an individual should always bow when facing a chamomile plant. This respect results from hundreds of years' experience with curing in folk medicine of the country.

Chamomile has been used for centuries to quiet an upset stomach, promote urination and relieve colic, and as a mild sleep aid. Topically, it has been used to reduce inflammation and soothe aches, and to heal cuts, sores, and bruises.

Current Status: Today's uses of chamomile differ little from those of ancient times. Chamomile is an official drug (recognized by government authority) in the pharmacopoeias of twenty-six countries. Anti-inflammatory, antiseptic, carminative, antispasmodic, and mild sedative activity as well as promotion of wound healing have been attributed to alpha-bisabolol, which comprises 13 percent of the essential oil. Another constituent, chamazulene, which comprises 5 percent of the essential oil, has been credited with relieving spasms, inflammation, pain, and allergy (but see "Cautions" on the next page).

In Europe, chamomile is used externally in compresses, rinses, or gargles; to treat inflammations and irritations of the skin and mucous membranes, including the mouth, gums, and respiratory tract; and for hemorrhoids. Chamomile tea or tincture relieves spasms and inflammation of the gastrointestinal tract as well as peptic ulcers. A mild tea makes a gentle sleep aid, particularly for children. Modern indications are backed not only by intensive recent research (except for sleep aid claims), but also by many centuries of common use.

Preparations: Dried flowers, herbal teas, capsules, salves, creams, tinctures, bath products, and other preparations are available in the American market.

Dosage: For tea, 2–3 g (½–1 tsp) of the dried flower are used three to four times daily. For tincture, 1–4 ml (10–40 drops) are used three times a day. For commercial preparations, follow label instructions. A soothing bath for hemorrhoids or skin irritation may be prepared by steeping up to a pound of flowers in 30 gallons of hot water.

Cautions: Persons who are allergic to the pollen of other members of the aster family, such as ragweed, may also be allergic to chamomile. Teas made from the dried flowers also contain pollen. Chamomile is associated with rare contact dermatitis. At least one case of anaphylactic shock has been attributed to drinking chamomile tea. Varro Tyler points out, however, that of fifty allergic reactions to "chamomiles" reported in the literature, only five were attributed to German chamomile, thus attesting to the herb's relative safety. Worldwide, approximately a million cups of chamomile tea are consumed daily.

Symptoms

Indigestion

Insomnia

Nausea

Actions

Anti-inflammatory

Promotes wound healing

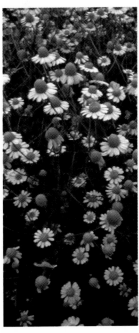

Cranberry

Vaccinium macrocarpon

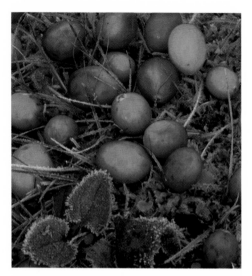

Source: A low-growing shrub of the heath family with leathery leaves and astringent red berries, cranberry is familiar to all, particularly in holiday sauces. It grows in bogs from Newfoundland to Manitoba south to Virginia, Ohio, and Illinois. Most of the commercial berries are produced in Massachusetts and Wisconsin.

Traditional Use: Cranberries and their juice have long been regarded as folk treatments for urinary infections. In early American medicine, the crushed berries were applied to tumors and poulticed on wounds. The berries were recognized as a treatment for scurvy (a vitamin C deficiency) and dysentery.

Current Status: Although cranberry has long been described as a urinary antiseptic, there is no convincing evidence that cranberry juice acidifies the urine to the point of inhibiting the growth of bacteria. Recently, however, scientists discovered that cranberry juice and extracts prevent adhesion of E. coli bacteria to linings of the bladder and the gut, inhibiting their ability to colonize and cause infection. A recent study of elderly patients found that drinking 4 to 6 ounces of cranberry juice daily had a preventative, rather than curative, effect on urinary tract infections. In other studies the juice was effective as a urinary deodorant in bedridden patients with high levels of white blood cells and bacteria in the urine.

Preparations: Cranberry is best known in the form of whole fruit, jelled fruit, and juice. Cranberry juice cocktail is a 33 percent dilution of pure juice with added sugars for flavoring. Cranberry is also available as dietary supplements in the form of dried fruit, fruit concentrates, and juice concentrate in 800-mg capsules.

Dosage: Five to 20 oz of cranberry juice cocktail daily (6 oz of juice is equal to 90 g of fresh fruit).

Cautions: If you suspect a urinary tract or kidney problem, see your doctor.

Symptoms

Urinary tract infections, mild

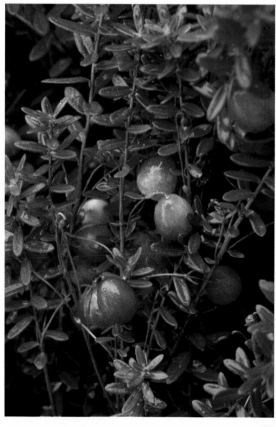

Dandelion

Taraxacum officinale

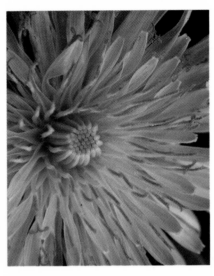

Source: Besides their culinary uses as coffee substitute and salad ingredient, the root and leaf of this pervasive weed of the aster family are also used in traditional medicine. Dandelion is grown commercially in both the United States and Europe.

Traditional Use: Both dandelion leaf and root have been used for centuries to treat liver, gall bladder, and kidney ailments, weak digestion, and rheumatism. They are also considered mildly laxative. The fresh root or its preparations are thought to be more potent than the dried root. The leaves have traditionally been used as a diuretic.

Current Status: Dandelion root and leaf are widely used in herbal medicines in Europe. The leaves are diuretic but also high in potassium, so they help to compensate for potassium lost with increased urination. Bitter compounds in the leaves (and root) increased bile secretion in laboratory animals by more than 40 percent. The leaves are prescribed as a diuretic in cases of water retention and for bloating accompanied by flatulence and loss of appetite.

The bitter compounds in dandelion root help stimulate digestion and are mildly laxative in activity. The roots have been shown to be moderately anti-inflammatory, which supports their traditional use in the treatment of rheumatism. The root is used for dyspepsia, loss of appetite, as a diuretic, and for disorders associated with inhibited bile secretion from the liver.

Preparations: The dried leaf and root, capsules, tinctures and tablets are available in the American market. Extracts (in 25 percent alcohol) are preferred for bile flow stimulation as the active compounds are more soluble in alcohol than in water.

Dosage: The dose of the dried leaf is 4–10 g, three times daily. The root is used in tea, with 1–2 tsp of the cut-and-sifted dried root steeped in a cup of hot water for 15 minutes. Take one cup in the morning and another in the evening.

Cautions: The German Commission E monographs on dandelion leaf and root indicate that in cases of gallstones, dandelion products should be used only under a physician's supervision. If bile ducts are obstructed, dandelion should not be used at all. The milky latex in fresh dandelion leaves may cause contact dermatitis. Bitter herbs such as dandelion root may also cause hyperacidity in some individuals.

Actions

Appetite stimulant
Diuretic
Increases bile flow

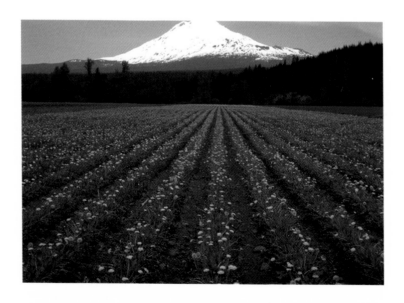

Dong-quai

Angelica sinensis

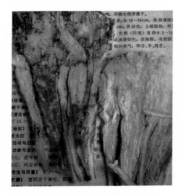

Source: Dong-quai is the dried root of a member of the parsley family. The plant thrives in high, cool, shaded mountain woods in south and western China. Most of the supply is commercially grown there, rather than wild-harvested.

Traditional Use: The name *dong-quai,* or *dang-gui,* means "proper order". Used in China for thousands of years, it is as highly regarded as ginseng. In traditional Chinese medicine (TCM), the root is believed to nourish the blood and help harmonize vital energy, thus returning the system to proper order. In China it is one of the more frequently prescribed herbs and appears in prescriptions (with other herbs) for abnormal or suppressed menstruation, anemia, and other conditions. In the West, it is used to tone and regulate the female reproductive system and is prescribed for premenstrual syndrome (PMS), menstrual difficulties, and menopause symptoms.

Current Status: Most research on the plant has been done in China and Japan since the early 1960s. Experiments show that whereas the volatile oil in the root causes relaxation of the uterine muscle, both water and alcohol extracts stimulate uterine contractions; alcohol extracts are stronger. Dong-quai also normalizes irregular uterine contractions, improving blood flow to the uterus. The actions do not appear to result from estrogenic activity, as dong-quai does not produce changes in the ovaries or vaginal tissue. It has been shown to improve circulation and lower blood pressure by increasing blood flow in the peripheral vessels and reducing vascular resistance. Experiments have also confirmed that it reduces inflammation, pain, and spasms, and increases the numbers of red blood cells and platelets. Animal studies have also confirmed that dong-quai protects the liver from toxins and helps it to utilize more oxygen. As most clinical studies in China and Japan have involved dong-quai in combination with other herbs, their generally positive results in treating gynecological problems are difficult to assess for dong-quai alone.

Preparations: Whole dried root, sliced root, powdered root, capsules, tablets, tinctures and combination products are all commonly available in the American market.

Dosage: In TCM, the root is made into a tea, or simmered to ½ the original volume of liquid, in doses of 5.4–12 g (1–3 tsp) per day.

Cautions: Pregnant or nursing women should avoid dong-quai unless under supervision of a qualified medical practitioner. In TCM, it is not given to patients with diarrhea, as it is considered somewhat laxative. Some angelica species are associated with contact dermatitis and related members of the parsley family are known to cause photodermatitis.

Symptoms

Menstrual difficulties
Menopausal difficulties
PMS

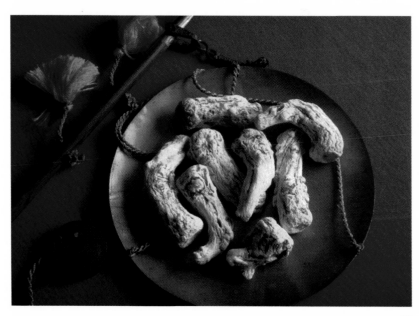

Echinacea

Echinacea angustifolia, E. pallida, E. purpurea

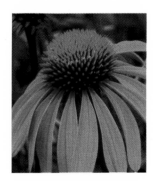

Sources: Echinacea, also known as purple coneflower, is the root or aboveground parts (harvested in flower) of three species of large, robust daisylike plants of the aster family. *Echinacea angustifolia* and *E. pallida* are harvested from the prairies of the midwestern United States. Some commercial cultivation of these two species has developed as they become more scarce in the wild. *E. purpurea,* also native to the Midwest, is the most widely used species of the three. The entire world supply is cultivated.

Traditional use: Native Americans of the prairie used echinacea for more medicinal purposes than they did any other plant, for everything from colds to cancer. It entered formal medicine in 1895, becoming the best-selling American medicinal plant prescribed by physicians into the 1920s. Later replaced by antibiotics in the United States, it has enjoyed continuous popularity in Europe. In 1993 German physicians prescribed echinacea more than 2.5 million times. Traditionally, herbalists consider it a blood purifier and aid to fighting infections.

Current Status: Today most consumers use echinacea to prevent and treat colds and to help heal infections. Echinacea enhances the particle ingestion capacity of white blood cells and other specialized immune system cells, thus increasing their ability to attack foreign invaders, such as cold or flu viruses. Besides stimulating a healthy immune system to deal more effectively with invading viruses, it helps accelerate healing if infection already exists.

A 1992 German double-blind, placebo-controlled study of 180 volunteers found that a dose of 4 droppers of tincture (equivalent to 900 mg of dried root) of *E. purpurea* root decreased symptoms and duration of flulike infections. More clinical studies are needed to determine clear therapeutic indications, the best preparations, and the most effective dosage. The best-studied echinacea is a preparation made from the fresh expressed juice of *E. purpurea.* No single chemical component has been identified as causing echinacea's medicinal action, but it may involve flavonoids, essential oils, polysaccharides, caffeic acid derivatives, alkylamides, and other compounds.

Preparations: Echinacea products include tablets, capsules, flex-tabs, and liquids such as tinctures, extracts, and the expressed juice of the fresh flowering plant, on which most research has been done. Some products are standardized to echinacoside, a derivative of caffeic acid, but this compound may not be involved in stimulation of the immune system.

Dosage: A dose of 60 drops of *E. purpurea* root tincture three times a day is equivalent to 1 g of the dried root three times a day. Rather than being used continuously like vitamin C to prevent colds, echinacea is used as needed at the onset of symptoms or in early stages of infection, usually for two weeks, followed by a resting period of one week.

Cautions: Persons who are allergic to the pollen of other members of the aster family, such as ragweed, may also be allergic to echinacea. The German government recommends that nonspecific immunostimulants, including echinacea, should not be used in cases of impaired immune response (involving diseases of the immune system itself) including tuberculosis, multiple sclerosis, and HIV infection.

Symptoms

Colds

Flu

Infections, minor

Actions

Prevents or reduces cold symptoms

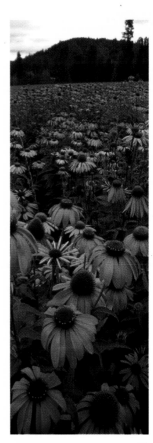

Eleuthero

Eleutherococcus senticosus

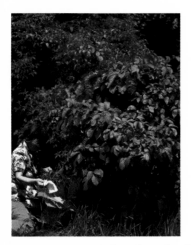

Source: Eleuthero, also known as Siberian ginseng, is the root, root bark, or stem of a shrub in the ginseng family. It grows in thickets in northeast China, eastern Russia, Korea, and Japan's northern island, Hokkaido. Most of the supply comes from Siberia and China, but it is also grown in eastern Europe. The Chinese call it *ci-wu-jia*.

Traditional Use: Eleuthero has been used in China as a tonic for invigorating vital energy (*qi*) for more than 2,000 years. It is listed in the first (most important) class of herbs in *Shen Nong Ben Cao Jing,* but some Chinese scholars question whether Shen Nong actually described eleuthero or another plant. Its recent use in China derives from Russian research since the early 1950s. In Chinese medicine, it is used to normalize body functions, restore vigor, improve health, promote good appetite, and help to assure a long life. Generally, it serves as a preventive medicine and general tonic.

Current Status: I. I. Brekhman, the leading Russian researcher on ginseng, has described eleuthero as an "adaptogen", an innocuous substance that causes minimal disorders of an organism's function. It must have a "nonspecific action" that normalizes body functions, no matter what the condition or disease. Adaptogens are essentially general tonics.

Since the early 1950s, studies have shown that eleuthero extract increases mental alertness, work output, and the quality of work under stressful conditions and in athletic performance. In addition, it strongly stimulates the immune system.

German authorities allow eleuthero to be labeled as an invigorating tonic for fatigue, convalescence, decreased work capacity, or difficulty in concentration.

Eleuthero

Preparations: In the United States, product forms include the dried powdered roots or stems, capsules, tablets, and tinctures. Most Russian research was done on a 33 percent ethanol extract.

Dose: Capsules in the United States typically contain 400–500 mg of the powdered root, with two capsules taken three times a day, equivalent to 2–3 g of the root per day.

In Russian studies involving healthy or stressed individuals, volunteers were given 2–16 ml of the extract one to three times daily for up to two months, followed by a two to three week resting period. This regimen was repeated up to five times in a year.

Cautions: Although no side effects, as such, are reported for eleuthero, the German Commission E notes that people with high blood pressure should avoid it, but there does not appear to be good clinical evidence to support this caution.

Actions

Adaptogen (tonic)

Immunostimulant

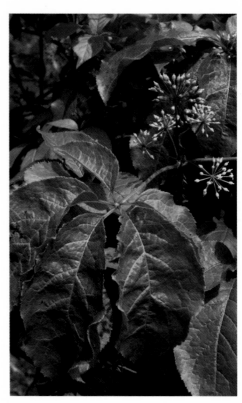

Ephedra

Ephedra sinica, E. intermedia, E. equisetina

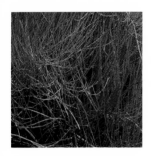

Sources: The Chinese herb *ma-huang,* known in the West as ephedra, is the dried stem of three species of primitive shrubs in the ephedra family found in desert regions around the world. Three species are commonly used as source plants: *E. sinica, E. intermedia,* and *E. equisetina,* all native to the steppes of north and northwestern China. The nine species and two hybrids that are native to North American deserts do not contain the alkaloids associated with the Asian species.

Traditional Use: Ma-huang is first mentioned in *Shen Nong Ben Cao Jing,* which survives as a list of 365 herbs from the first century A.D. In traditional Chinese medicine (TCM) its functions are to induce sweat, soothe breath, and promote urination. It is prescribed for bad colds, fevers without sweat, pain in the joints, coughing, shortness of breath, and swelling of the ankles. Ephedra has been used for more than 2,000 years to treat bronchial asthma, colds and flu, chills, lack of perspiration, headache, nasal congestion, aching joints and bones, cough and wheezing, and edema.

Current Status: The basis of ephedra's medicinal use is its alkaloids ephedrine and pseudoephedrine, which stimulate the central nervous system and heart muscle, dilate the bronchial tubes, and elevate blood pressure. Both natural ephedrine and pseudoephedrine from ma-huang and synthetic forms of the alkaloids are sold commercially. Pseudoephedrine's effects are somewhat weaker than those of ephedrine. Ephedra also has diuretic and anti-inflammatory activity.

The alkaloids are used in over-the-counter bronchodilators for mild seasonal asthma or chronic asthma. They are also found in products to relieve sinusitis and nasal congestion.

Preparations: Ma-huang is available in crude form (dried stems) in the American market, and is formulated in teas, capsules, tablets, and other products. It is often inappropriately used in weight-loss products and stimulants. The alkaloids ephedrine and pseudoephedrine are ingredients in dozens of cold, allergy, and cough products.

Ephedra

Dose: The herb itself contains 1 percent or less of ephedrine and is used in TCM in a dose of 1.5–6 g in tea. Ephedrine is formulated in legitimate over-the-counter drug products in doses for adults of 12.5–25 mg every four hours. No more than 150 mg should be taken in 24 hours.

Cautions: A discussion of the side effects of this herb or its alkaloids when abused could fill a small book. Some of the known effects include insomnia, motor disturbances, high blood pressure, glaucoma, impaired cerebral circulation, and urinary disturbances. Ephedrine-containing products should not be used by anyone who has hypertension, high blood pressure, heart disease, thyroid disease or diabetes, or who is taking a monoamine oxidase inhibitor.

Over-the-counter drugs containing ephedra alkaloids are required to carry a warning against exceeding the recommended dose (except under a physician's direction). Also, if symptoms are not relieved in an hour or worsen, discontinue use immediately and seek a physician's advice. Abuse of ephedra alkaloid products has led to more than a dozen reported deaths, often due to heart failure. It is best to seek the opinion of a physician before using ephedra products.

Symptoms

Asthma, mild

Nasal congestion

Actions

Bronchodilator

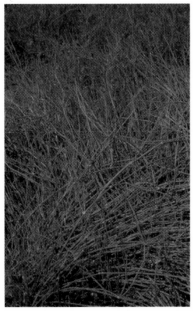

Evening primrose

Oenothera biennis

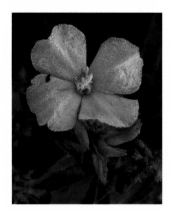

Source: Evening primrose oil is obtained from the seeds of a common wildflower of the evening primrose family native to eastern North America and widely naturalized in Europe and western North America. Most of the seed for oil production is grown commercially.

Traditional Use: Native Americans gathered the seeds for food in Utah and Nevada. Those in eastern North America used the whole plant as a poultice for bruises, a tea to treat obesity, and a decoction of the root to treat hemorrhoids. Early settlers used the leaves to treat wounds and to soothe sore throats and upset stomach. Use of the seed oil is relatively recent.

Current Status: Evening primrose oil has been used as a dietary supplement to provide essential fatty acids, especially gamma-linolenic acid (GLA). GLA is an intermediate compound between the essential fatty acid, cis-linoleic acid and prostaglandin production in the body. Factors such as aging, alcohol abuse, cancerous conditions, poor dietary habits, or improper nutrition may prevent the natural conversion of cis-linoleic acid into prostaglandin E_1. Dietary supplementation of GLA from evening primrose oil can help resolve problems associated with essential-fatty-acid deficiencies.

More than 120 studies in fifteen countries report potential use of the seed oil in treating imbalances and abnormalities of essential fatty acids, including allergy-induced eczema, asthma, migraine, inflammations, premenstrual syndrome (PMS), diabetes, arthritis, and alcoholism. Conflicting results point to the need for further well-designed scientific studies. For example, in some double-blind placebo-controlled clinical studies evening primrose oil significantly reduced breast pain and tenderness, irritability, and mood swings associated with PMS. Another clinical study, however, showed improvement in PMS symptoms from evening primrose oil, but when compared to placebo, the results were deemed statistically insignificant.

Evening primrose

Preparations: Evening primrose oil is available in 500-mg capsules.

Dose: Three to six capsules a day may be recommended, or as much as 6 g (twelve capsules). It should be taken with meals.

Cautions: No known contraindications or drug interactions have been reported for evening primrose oil. In clinical studies, fewer than 2 percent of patients taking it for long periods reported side effects such as abdominal discomfort, nausea, and headache.

Symptoms

Essential fatty acids deficiency

PMS

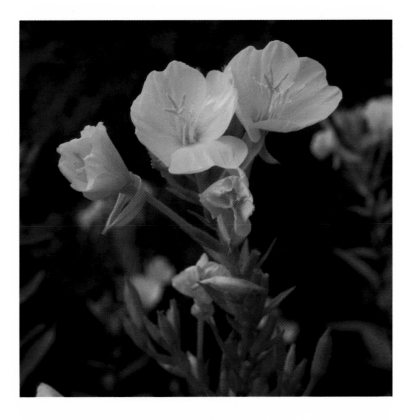

Feverfew

Tanacetum parthenium (formerly Chrysanthemum parthenium)

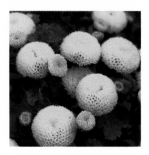

Source: Feverfew is the fresh or dried leaf of a member of the aster family native to the Balkan peninsula. It is naturalized in Europe, as well as in North and South America.

Traditional Use: The English herbalist Nicholas Culpeper (1787) wrote that feverfew "is very effectual for all pains in the head coming of a cold cause, the herb being bruised and applied to the crown of the head." For more than 2,000 years, feverfew was a folk medicine taken internally for fevers, headache, or menstrual regulation, or applied externally to relieve pain.

Current Status: Modern use focuses on feverfew to help prevent migraines. A compound called parthenolide (not found in all feverfew varieties) appears to be responsible for its antimigraine effects.

During the past decade, clinical interest in feverfew increased after an English newspaper asked for volunteers with experience in using feverfew for migraines and received 25,000 replies. Of three hundred volunteers, 70 percent claimed a reduction in migraine frequency or pain after eating one to three fresh leaves a day. In a 1985 double-blind study conducted by London researchers, seventeen patients ingested an average daily dose of 60 mg of feverfew leaves and experienced no change in frequency or severity of migraine symptoms. Those who took the placebo, however, had an increase in frequency and severity of headaches, nausea, and vomiting.

In a 1988 randomized, double-blind, placebo-controlled, crossover study on feverfew in migraine prevention in Nottingham, seventy-two volunteers received either a feverfew capsule or a placebo daily for four months. The feverfew treatment was associated with a reduction in frequency of migraine headaches and related vomiting as well as some reduction in migraine severity; the duration of migraine attacks was not significantly shortened.

Preparations: The fresh leaves, dried leaves, capsules standardized to parthenolide content, tablets, and tinctures are available in the American market. Canadian authorities have adopted a 0.2 percent parthenolide content as a minimum standard for feverfew products.

Dose: The average daily dose is calculated as 125 mg of dried leaves each day, assuming a minimum parthenolide content of 0.2 percent. This is equivalent to eating two average-sized fresh leaves each day.

Cautions: No long-term studies have been done on safety. Mouth ulcers have been reported in 7 to 12 percent of patients who chewed the fresh leaves; tongue inflammation, swelling of the lips, and occasional loss of taste sometimes prevent continued use. These symptoms disappear when use is stopped. Avoid during pregnancy.

Symptoms

Migraine headaches

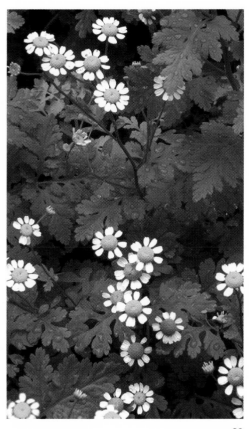

Fo-ti

Polygonum multiflorum

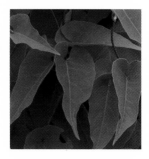

Source: Fo-ti is the dried or cured root of a twining vine in the knotweed family, found throughout China, except in the extreme northeast. It is also occasionally grown in American gardens as an ornamental. Ask Chinese herbalists about "fo-ti" and they won't know what you're talking about. The name was given to the plant by a marketer in the early 1970s for the American herb business. In China, it is known as *he-shou-wu*.

Traditional Use: In Chinese medicine the dried (unprocessed) root and the cured (processed) root are considered two different herbs. The unprocessed root is used to relax the bowels and detoxify the blood. The processed root is used to strengthen the blood, invigorate the liver and kidneys, and supplement vital energy (*qi*). Processed fo-ti is one of the more widely used tonics in traditional Chinese medicine (TCM), which employs it to enhance longevity, increase vigor, and promote fertility. It is also an ingredient in TCM formulas for premature gray hair, low back pain, angina pectoris, low energy, and other conditions.

Current Status: In animals, the processed root reduces blood cholesterol. The root contains lectins, which appear to help prevent cholesterol accumulation in the liver and fat retention in the blood. Animal experiments show it can help reduce formation of plaque and fat deposits on arterial walls. Fo-ti also inhibits the growth of bacteria, increases laboratory animals' ability to adapt to cold temperatures, and promotes the formation of red blood cells. An extract of the processed root has also shown antitumor, antioxidant, and immunostimulant effects in animals. Unprocessed roots lubricate the bowels, producing a laxative effect. Several clinical studies in China suggest the processed herb is useful in treating high cholesterol, heart conditions, and chronic bronchitis. Mounting evidence supports fo-ti's traditional use as a tonic.

Preparations: The whole root, sliced root, root powder, capsules, tablets, and tinctures are found in the American market, mostly in tonics. Unfortunately, few American herb books (and even the scientific literature) make a distinction between the unprocessed and processed forms of the roots. The processed forms have been boiled in a special black bean liquid according to traditional methods. This "curing" process changes the action of the root. Most American products contain the cheaper unprocessed root, which is mildly laxative. The unprocessed root is light brown to brown in color while the processed or cured root is dark reddish brown.

Dose: In TCM, 6–15 g (1 tsp–1 tbsp) of the dried root are simmered in teas with other herbs. For products in the American market, follow the label instructions.

Cautions: The unprocessed root can cause loose stools or diarrhea, sometimes with intestinal pain and nausea. The unprocessed root is considered potentially more toxic than the processed form. One case of allergic reaction to the cured root has been reported, although this form of fo-ti is considered to be minimally toxic when taken in proper doses. Large doses have resulted in numbness of the extremities as well as skin rashes.

Actions

Adaptogen (tonic)
Blood-builder
Lowers cholesterol

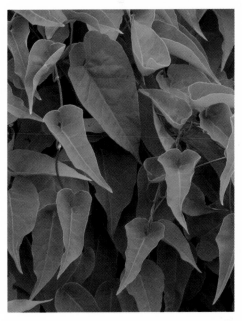

Garlic

Allium sativum

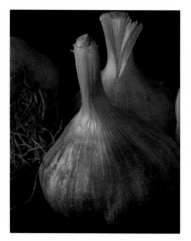

Source: No herb is so closely tied to the human experience as garlic. The bulb of a member of the lily family, it is unknown from the wild. Garlic has actually evolved under cultivation during the past 5,000 years.

Traditional Use: Garlic has been used as food and medicine since the age of the Egyptian pharaohs. The Greek historian and traveler Herodotus (484–425 B.C.) wrote that inscriptions on an Egyptian pyramid recorded the quantities of garlic consumed by the laborers. The Roman naturalist Pliny the Elder (A.D. 23–79) declared, "Garlic has powerful properties, and is of great benefit against changes of water and of residence." He recommended it to treat asthma, suppress coughs, and expel intestinal parasites, but noted some drawbacks (other than garlic breath): garlic dulled the sight, caused flatulence, injured the stomach if taken in excess, and caused thirst. In China, garlic was traditionally used for fevers, dysentery and intestinal parasites. Its antibacterial activity was first recognized in an 1858 study by the French microbiologist Louis Pasteur.

Current Status: In the past twenty years garlic has been the subject of more than 2,500 credible scientific studies. Well-documented health benefits include reducing cholesterol and triglycerides in the blood (while increasing high-density lipoproteins, so-called good cholesterol), reducing blood pressure, improving circulation, and helping to prevent yeast infections, cancers, colds, and flu. Garlic has good antibacterial, antifungal, antiparasitic, antioxidant, anti-inflammatory, and immunostimulant properties. At least nine epidemiological studies show that garlic significantly decreases the incidence of cancer, especially cancers of the gastrointestinal tract, among those who consume it regularly.

When garlic is cut or crushed, it produces sulfur compounds, such as allicin, because a sulfur-containing amino acid, alliin, comes into

Garlic

contact with the enzyme allinase. Garlic has an extremely complex chemistry, with more than 160 compounds identified from its bulbs and essential oil.

If your food should be your medicine, garlic should be part of your diet.

Preparations: Garlic is available in many product forms, including, of course, fresh and dried garlic, as well as capsules, "odorless" garlic tablets, and aged garlic extracts.

Dose: One average-sized clove of fresh garlic may be chewed daily as a general preventive. Add raw garlic to cooked foods at the end of cooking to retain sulfur compounds and volatile constituents. According to German health authorities, the daily dose is 4 g of fresh garlic. Processed garlic products should deliver at least 5,000 micrograms of allicin daily. Clinical and pharmacological studies since 1988 show that 900 mg of powdered garlic standardized to 0.6 percent allicin per 100 mg (equivalent to 5.4 mg allicin) daily can lower cholesterol.

Cautions: Rare cases of allergic reactions to garlic have been reported. Some individuals experience heartburn or flatulence from consuming it.

Actions

Chemopreventive

Lowers cholesterol

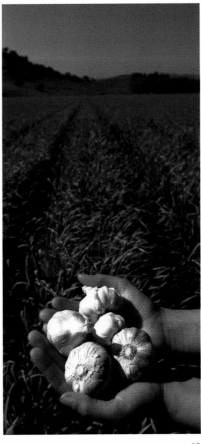

Ginger

Zingiber officinale

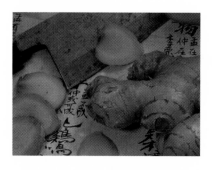

Source: Ginger is the dried or fresh root of a tropical member of the ginger family native to the Old World tropics.

Traditional Use: Cultivated for millennia in both China and India, ginger reached the West at least 2,000 years ago. Most of the thousands of prescriptions in Chinese traditional medicine (TCM) are combinations of many herbs; ginger is used in nearly half of them to mediate the effects of other ingredients as well as to stimulate the appetite and calm the stomach. In European herbal traditions, ginger is primarily used to stop nausea and quiet an upset stomach.

Current Status: Ginger is now recognized for helping to treat stomach upset and prevent symptoms of motion sickness. It has been studied for its antibacterial, antifungal, pain-relieving, anti-ulcer, antitumor, and other properties. Six clinical studies have looked at ginger's potential to reduce motion sickness. Four European studies reported positive results, while two American studies gave negative findings. In one English study, thirty-six volunteers were given either ginger or a common anti-motion sickness drug. When blindfolded and subjected to time in a spinning chair, those who took ginger held out an average of 5.5 minutes, while those who took the conventional drug lasted about 3.5 minutes before becoming ill. Another study involved eighty naval cadets at sea. Those who took a placebo developed seasickness. Those who were given gingerroot capsules had fewer cold sweats and less nausea. A 1988 NASA study that tested ginger in forty-two volunteers, however, concluded it was ineffective in relieving motion sickness. Clearly, more studies are needed.

Ginger is believed to reduce nausea by increasing digestive fluids and absorbing and neutralizing toxins and stomach acid. It increases bile secretion as well as the action and tone of the bowel. Ginger also has been shown to reduce the stickiness of blood platelets and may thereby reduce the risk of atherosclerosis. Limited studies suggest ginger may reduce morning sickness as well as nausea after surgery. Both

Ginger

uses require a physician's supervision.

Preparations: Fresh root, dried root, capsules, tablets, tinctures, and standardized products. The dried roots have a synergistic interaction between compounds in the essential oil and pungent principles such as gingerol. Some products are now standardized to gingerol content.

Dose: Two to 4 g ($\frac{1}{2}$ to 1 tsp) of dried root are divided into three portions as an average daily dose. Follow label instructions on standardized products.

Cautions: The German therapeutic monograph on ginger warns patients with gall bladder disease to avoid it and also cautions against exceeding the recommend dosage. Pregnant women contemplating ginger use during morning sickness (short-term only) should avoid it if gall bladder disease is present.

Symptoms

Indigestion
Motion sickness
Nausea

Actions

Digestive stimulant

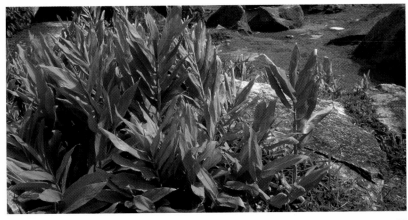

Ginkgo

Ginkgo biloba

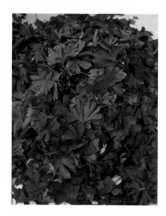

Sources: Ginkgo products come from the leaves of the only surviving member of the ginkgo family, a living fossil more than 200 million years old. Most commercial leaf production is from plantations in South Carolina, France, and China.

Traditional Use: Ginkgo leaf is a relatively new herbal medicine, used in China only since the fifteenth century. The leaves were traditionally used for "benefiting the brain", treatment of lung disorders, relief of cough and asthma symptoms, and diarrhea. The leaf tea was applied externally to treat sores of the skin and remove freckles.

Current Status: Ginkgo leaf extracts are among the better-selling herbal medicines in Europe. Most research has focused on the use of the complex extracts to increase circulation to the extremities as well as the brain, especially in the elderly. Clinical use is supported by more than 400 scientific studies conducted since the late 1950s. Ginkgo extract has also been studied for the treatment of ringing in the ears (tinnitus), male impotence, degenerative nerve conditions such as multiple sclerosis, and other diseases. It has shown potential to relieve difficulties with short-term memory, attention span, and mood in early stages of Alzheimer's disease by improving oxygen metabolism in the brain.

Ginkgo's effects have been attributed to compounds called flavone glycosides, as well as unique compounds—ginkgolides—which are potent inhibitors of a platelet-activating factor involved in the development of inflammatory, cardiovascular, and respiratory disorders. The ginkgolides' activity helps explain the herb's broad-spectrum biological effects.

Another important effect is strong antioxidant activity. With its ability to "scavenge" reactive oxygen forms known as free radicals, ginkgo leaf extract directs antioxidant effects to the brain, central nervous system, and cardiovascular system. This is one of the mechanisms that make it promising in treatment of age-related declines of brain function.

Preparations: Ginkgo is one of the few herbs produced in very complex forms with predictable effects. Nearly all studies have been conducted on a highly concentrated ginkgo leaf extract standardized to 24 percent flavone glycosides, further calibrated for six percent ginkgolides, and with potentially toxic ginkgolic acid removed. The results of studies on the complex leaf extract do not apply to the dried leaf or leaf tea.

Dose: For predictable results with standardized ginkgo leaf products, the dose is very specific and cannot be translated into kitchen measures. Typical dosage ranges for ginkgo leaf extract are 120–160 mg daily (divided into three doses). Some German physicians prescribe 240 mg daily doses. Ginkgo is generally used for six to eight weeks before results are evident.

Cautions: Some individuals have shown hypersensitivity to ginkgo leaf extracts including rare cases of gastrointestinal upset, headaches, or skin allergies. In such cases, use of ginkgo should be discontinued.

Symptoms

Age-related memory loss

Tinnitus

Actions

Antioxidant

Improves microcirculation

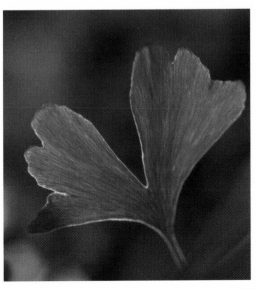

Ginseng

Panax quinquefolius, P. ginseng

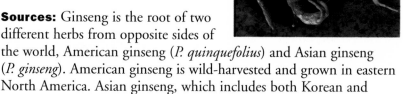

Sources: Ginseng is the root of two different herbs from opposite sides of the world, American ginseng (*P. quinquefolius*) and Asian ginseng (*P. ginseng*). American ginseng is wild-harvested and grown in eastern North America. Asian ginseng, which includes both Korean and Chinese ginseng, is cultivated in China, Korea, and Japan.

Traditional Use: According to the Harvard University botanist Shiu Ying Hu, the earliest mention of ginseng is in the 2,000-year-old herbal of Shen Nong:

> It is used for repairing the five viscera, quieting the spirit, curbing the emotion, stopping agitation, removing noxious influence, brightening the eyes, enlightening the mind and increasing wisdom. Continuous use leads one to longevity with light weight.

Ginseng use has changed little in 2,000 years.

Current Status: In the last thirty years, Asian ginseng (but not American ginseng) has been extensively studied. Like eleuthero, ginseng is an adaptogen. At least seven European clinical studies showed that standardized extracts decreased reaction time to visual and auditory stimuli; increased respiratory performance, alertness, power of concentration, and grasp of abstract concepts; and improved visual and motor coordination. Sometimes conflicting results indicate the need for further clinical studies, especially on products with well-defined levels of active compounds.

Recent studies have focused on antiviral and metabolic effects, antioxidant activity, and effects on nervous and reproductive systems. Ginseng is also a nonspecific immunostimulant similar to echinacea.

There are more than eighteen active chemicals called ginsenosides in Asian ginseng. American and Asian ginsengs contain some of the same as well as some different ginsenosides which explains their different actions as expressed in traditional Chinese medicine (TCM). Mild American ginseng helps to reduce the heat of the respiratory and digestive systems, whereas the stronger Asian ginseng is a heat-raising tonic for the blood and circulatory systems.

In Germany, Asian ginseng products may be labeled as tonics to treat fatigue, reduced work capacity, lack of concentration, and convalescence.

Ginseng

Preparations: Asian ginseng is available as whole root, powder, and in various forms including "white" and "red" ginseng. White ginseng is simply the dried root; translucent, rust-colored "red" ginseng is made by steaming the roots for three hours, then drying them; it is considered stronger than white ginseng. Product forms include tinctures, capsules, tablets, teas, and extracts. Asian ginseng products standardized to contain 4–7 percent ginsenosides are widely sold and may produce more reliable effects than other forms. American ginseng is generally available as the whole or powdered root.

Dose: The German Commission E monograph on ginseng recommends a daily dosage of 1–2 g of Asian ginseng root, divided into three portions. TCM prescribes 1–9 g of Asian ginseng or 2–9 g of American ginseng. Higher dosages may be prescribed by health care practitioners as needed. For standardized products, 100 mg one or two times a day is the usual recommended dose.

Cautions: Use at normal dosage levels is generally not associated with side effects; however, some persons have experienced overstimulation or gastrointestinal upset and some women have reported breast tenderness or menstrual problems with long-term use. If you have high blood pressure, use ginseng with caution. Avoid ginseng during pregnancy.

Symptoms

Convalescence

Fatigue

Actions

Adaptogen (tonic)

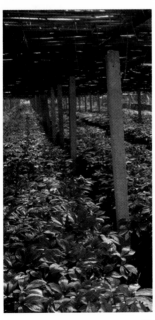

Goldenseal

Hydrastis canadensis

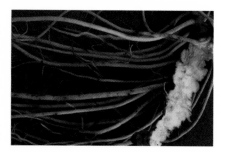

Source: Goldenseal is the root and rhizome of a member of the buttercup family. It grows in rich woods from Vermont to Georgia, west to Alabama and Arkansas, north to eastern Iowa and Minnesota.

Traditional Use: The Cherokee used the roots topically to treat inflammations and drank a root tea to improve appetite and for dyspepsia. The Iroquois used it for liver disorders, fever, sour stomach, and diarrhea.

Goldenseal was listed among the official remedies in the first revision (1830) of the New York edition of the *U. S. Pharmacopoeia*. It was dropped in 1840, then listed again from 1860 to 1926. The root was used primarily for inflammations of the mucous membranes.

Current Status: Goldenseal is one of the more popular American herbs. It is used as an antiseptic, to stop bleeding, and as a tonic and anti-inflammatory for the mucous membranes. Components derived from the root have been used in eyewashes.

In the past century, very little scientific research has been done on goldenseal. Its major effects are attributed to the alkaloids hydrastine and berberine. In animal experiments, hydrastine lowered blood pressure; berberine stimulated digestion and the secretion of bile, lowered blood pressure, and inhibited growth of bacteria. Berberine gives goldenseal its yellow color and bitter taste.

One modern folk use of goldenseal is based on the plot of a 1900 novel by the pharmacist John Uri Lloyd, *Stringtown on the Pike:* ingesting the herb in an attempt to mask the presence of illicit drugs in the urine. Although there is no scientific evidence to support this practice, some laboratories now test for goldenseal in urinalysis. Still widely used, goldenseal is a plant in need of new research.

Preparations: The whole and powdered dried root is available, as is the leaf, which contains some of the root alkaloids but in smaller concentrations. Capsules, tablets, tinctures, extracts, salves, and ointments are also available.

Dose: *The British Herbal Compendium* lists a daily dose of ½–1 g (a pinch) of the powdered root divided into three doses or 2–4 ml (20–40 drops) of tincture made from one part root to ten parts 60 percent ethanol solution.

Cautions: Fresh goldenseal may cause ulcerations of the skin when applied externally; reports of this reaction relate to homeopathic remedies of the mid-nineteenth century which contained jimsonweed and zinc oxide in addition to goldenseal. No recent reports of toxicity occur in the literature. Several books warn pregnant and nursing women and people with heart problems to use goldenseal cautiously, presumably because of the lack of toxicity studies. While it has not been documented scientifically, goldenseal may disrupt intestinal flora; some herbalists therefore recommend taking acidophilus with it.

Symptoms

Inflammation of mucous membranes

Actions

Antibacterial

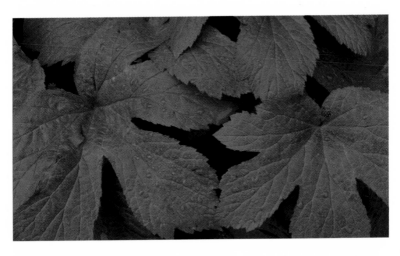

Gotu kola

Centella asiatica (formerly *Hydrocotyle asiatica*)

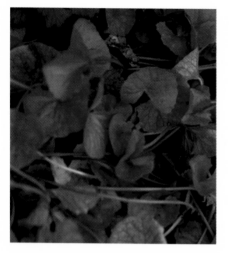

Source: Gotu kola is a low-growing herb in the parsley family native to tropical Asia, where it is grown commercially. It also grows in Hawaii and other tropical regions.

Traditional Use: In India, the ancient tradition of Ayurveda regards gotu kola as an important rejuvenating herb, especially for nerve and brain cells. It is prescribed to increase intelligence, longevity, and memory while retarding senility and aging. A leaf tea is used as a wash for skin diseases, inflammation, and swelling. In Chinese folk medicine, the leaf tea is used for colds, lung and urinary tract infections, and externally for snakebite, injuries, and shingles.

Current Status: The notion that gotu kola promotes intelligence led to a number of studies of its effect on the central nervous system. Preliminary results showed it can be beneficial in improving memory and may also help overcome stress and fatigue. Two older Indian studies reported that it helped improve intelligence, general mental abilities, and behavior in mentally retarded children.

A later study examined how the herb affected brain neurotransmitters in laboratory rats. For two weeks, some rats were given an extract of fresh gotu kola leaves. They scored three to sixty times better than untreated rats in tests of learning and memory. A decrease of neurotransmitters was correlated with their improved learning and memory.

Other experiments indicate that gotu kola acts as a mild depressant on the central nervous system. Topically, it relieves-inflammation, strengthens tissue at wound sites, and helps rebuild damaged skin tissue. In one clinical study of a topical preparation of gotu kola, thirteen of twenty patients with poorly healing wounds experienced complete, accelerated healing.

Preparations: Gotu kola is available in the American market as dried cut-and-sifted or powdered herb in tea, capsules, tablets, and tinctures. Salves and ointments, standardized to asiaticoside, are available in other countries to treat wounds.

Dose: An average daily dose is 600 mg of the dried powdered leaves in capsules, or use 1 tsp of the dried herb in a cup of hot water to make tea.

Cautions: None noted.

Symptoms

Cuts and abrasions

Stress

Actions

Improves memory

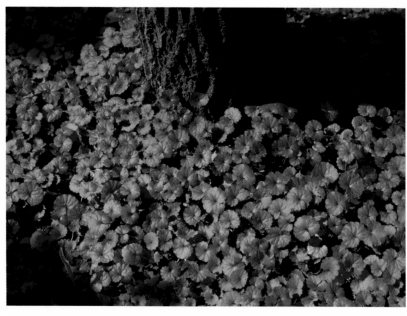

Hawthorn

Crataegus spp.

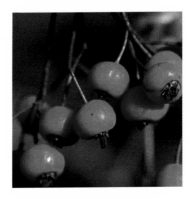

Sources: Hawthorn is the fruit, or the flowers and leaves combined, of several of the more than 100 species of *Crataegus*, a genus of the rose family found in North America, Europe, and east Asia.

In Europe, English hawthorn, *C. laevigata,* and oneseed hawthorn, *C. monogyna* are used. In Chinese medicine, *C. pinnatifida* is used.

Traditional Use: If closely related plants are used by cultures on opposite sides of the globe, a scientific basis for the traditional use is likely. Such is the case with hawthorns, which have been used in European, Chinese, and American traditions alike to treat heart ailments. In traditional Asian medicine as well as European herbal traditions, hawthorn has been widely used in long-term prescriptions for hypertension related to cardiac weakness, arteriosclerosis, and angina pectoris.

Hawthorn is notably absent from medical works and herbals of early-nineteenth-century America and Europe. It came to the attention of the medical profession in the 1890s by means of a single reference in a medical journal. By the early twentieth century, it was a mainstay of heart disease treatment. Still widely used in Europe and Asia, it is less frequently recommended in America.

Current Status: Medical practitioners in Europe and China use hawthorn to treat early stages of congestive heart failure characterized by diminished cardiac function, a sensation of pressure or anxiety in the heart area, age-related heart disorders which do not require digitalis, and mild arrhythmias. Numerous pharmacological and clinical studies have shown that hawthorn fruit or berry extract improves blood flow to and from the heart by strengthening its contractions. Hawthorn flower and leaf extracts improve circulation to the extremities by reducing resistance in the arteries. Experiments in China have shown that preparations of hawthorn fruit lower blood pressure and serum cholesterol levels, and are therefore useful in the prevention and treatment of arteriosclerosis.

Preparations: Preparations used in Europe are standardized to compounds called oligomeric procyanidins and flavonoids. The dried berries, leaves, and flowers are available in the American market. Standardized products may be expected to give more predictable results. The berries also make a pleasant-tasting tea. In Germany flower and leaf preparations are approved. Fruit preparations are unapproved since they are not as extensively researched as flower and leaf preparations.

Dose: The usual dose is 160 mg per day divided in two portions. Under a physician's supervision, as much as 160 mg three times daily may be prescribed in Europe. Traditionally, a tea is made from 4–5 g of the fruits.

Cautions: No side effects or contraindications are known from hawthorn. Any heart condition, however, is serious and should receive the attention of qualified medical practitioners. Heart disease is the number one killer in America; it should not be self-diagnosed or self-treated.

Symptoms

Angina pectoris

Congestive heart failure, early stages

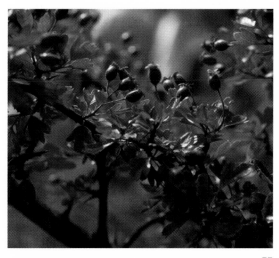

Hops

Humulus lupulus

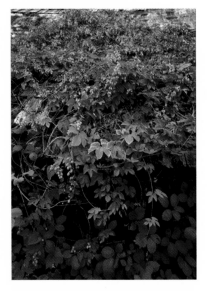

Source: Hops are the fruiting bodies or strobiles of a member of the cannabis family native to Europe, Asia, and North America. Hops are widely grown in the Pacific Northwest, primarily for flavoring beer. They are also cultivated in Germany; the Czech Republic is famous for its high quality hops.

Traditional Use: Traditionally, hops were considered soothing to the stomach, an appetite stimulant (due to the bitter taste), slightly sedative, a sleep aid, and diuretic. A popular way of using hops as a sleep aid was to stuff a pillow with the fruiting bodies, moistening them slightly before bed to prevent them from rustling and keeping an insomniac awake! A poultice of hops was used to relieve pain of rheumatic joints and a tea was taken to relieve muscle spasms and soothe the nerves.

Current Status: In European phytomedicine, hops preparations are used to relieve mood disturbances, such as unrest and anxiety, and for sleep disturbances. Hops are also prescribed for nervous tension, excitability, restlessness and lack of sleep, and to stimulate appetite. Laboratory studies show that hops have a wide range of biological activity. The bitter acids in the fruits are antibacterial. Extracts of the fruits strongly reduce smooth-muscle spasms. Studies have both confirmed and disputed hops' sedative and estrogenic activities.

Preparations: The dried fruits (strobiles), from which a tea can be made, are commonly available, as are tinctures, capsules, and tablets. Hops are often used in combination with other sleep aids or calming herbs such as valerian, passionflower, or skullcap.

Dose: German health authorities recommend a daily dose of only ½ g. That may be more than you think, however, because hops are very light in weight. Use about 1 heaping tsp of whole hops to make tea.

Cautions: No side effects, contraindications, or adverse drug interactions from the use of hops are generally reported, though some individuals have experienced a rare allergic reaction or contact dermatitis from the pollen or the yellow powder-like crystals in the fruits.

Symptoms

Anxiety

Insomnia

Lack of appetite

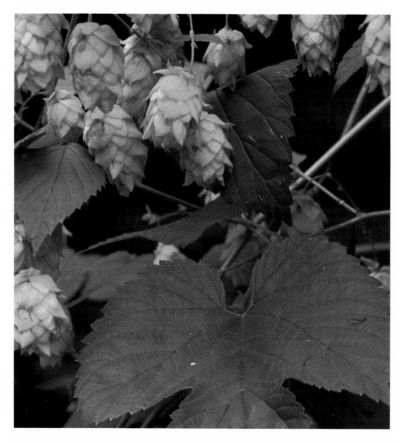

Kava-kava

Piper methysticum

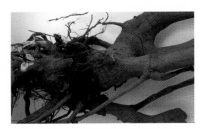

Source: Kava-kava, or simply kava, as it is also known, is the massive root stock or leaf of a highly variable sprawling shrub in the pepper family, found throughout the South Pacific islands from Hawaii to New Guinea. The plant has been cultivated for so many centuries that its exact origin is unclear. Like garlic, kava in its present form evolved during 3,000 years of cultivation.

Traditional Use: Polynesians have used a thick brew of the fresh or dried root as their main beverage for centuries. A similar beverage, prepared from ground roots, is often imbibed in social or ceremonial settings. The cultural role of kava in Pacific societies has been compared to that of wine in southern Europe. A decoction of the rootstock has reportedly been used for the treatment of gonorrhea, chronic cystitis and other urinary infections, menstrual problems, migraine headache, insomnia, and other conditions.

The first herb products made from kava appeared in Europe in the 1860s. By the 1890s, kava extracts were available in German herb shops. The first pharmaceutical preparation, a tincture used as a mild sedative and to lower blood pressure, became available in Germany thirty years later.

Current Status: In Germany the rootstock and its preparations are allowed to be labeled for conditions of nervous anxiety, stress, and unrest. In Europe, kava extracts are often combined with pumpkin seed, for its diuretic effect, in the treatment of irritable bladder syndrome.

Compounds called kavalactones give kava root its primary effects. Two of them, in specified dosages, have pain-relieving effects comparable to aspirin. One kavalactone produces a numbing effect in the mouth upon chewing the root or drinking kava preparations. Kavalactones have been shown to relax muscles by affecting muscular contractility rather than by blocking neurotransmitter signals in nerves.

Preparations: Kava root tablets, capsules, tinctures, and dried root are available in the American market as are kava leaf products. Standardized European products contain 70 percent kavalactones.

Dose: Standardized extracts used in clinical studies have a dosage of 100 mg per day divided into three portions. Otherwise, follow label instructions. Do not exceed dosage.

Cautions: The German health authorities warn that kava should not be used during pregnancy, lactation, or depression. Because of its apparent sedative action, it should not be taken with alcohol, or when operating machinery or vehicles. No side effects are associated with small amounts of kava preparations. In the copious amounts consumed on South Sea islands, side effects of long-term use include temporary yellow discoloration of the skin, hair, and nails; rare allergic skin reactions; and vision disturbances. Excessive use has also caused skin itching and sores. In some Western popular articles and books, kava has been described as a "hypnotic", but, contrary to the wishful thinking of some promoters, it is neither hallucinogenic, nor stupefying, nor does it produce any physical addiction.

Symptoms

Anxiety

Insomnia

Stress

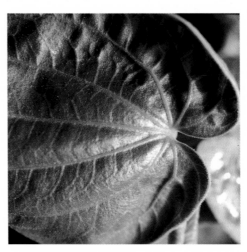

Lemon balm

Melissa officinalis

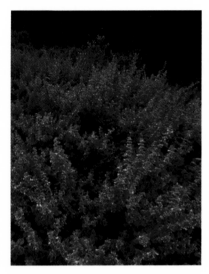

Source: Lemon balm is the leaf of a perennial herb in the mint family native to the Mediterranean region, western Asia, southwestern Siberia, and northern Africa. It is widely naturalized in North America and elsewhere.

Traditional Use: Lemon balm's history dates back at least 2,000 years. It has been used to reduce fevers, induce sweating, calm the digestive tract, treat colds, and relieve spasms related to cramps and headaches. In medieval Europe, the tea was valued for disorders of the nervous system. It has long been a popular folk remedy for insomnia. Lemon balm was official in the *U. S. Pharmacopoeia* from 1840 to 1890.

Current Status: Lemon balm has been shown to be sedative, to relieve spasms, and inhibit the growth of fungi and bacteria. The German government allows preparations of lemon balm to be labeled for difficulty in falling asleep due to nervous conditions and for spasms of the digestive tract.

Laboratory experiments have shown activity against viruses including mumps and herpes simplex. A lemon balm cream is sold in Germany for cold sores and conditions related to herpes simplex. In a clinical study of 115 patients with herpes, a cream containing 1 percent dried lemon balm extract was applied by the patients as needed five times daily for up to fourteen days until healing of herpes lesions was complete. In 96 percent of the patients, lesions were healed by day eight of the treatment, in 87 percent by day six, and in 60 percent by day four. Unassisted healing usually takes ten to fourteen days. A subsequent randomized, placebo-controlled, double-blind study compared the effect of the same cream with a placebo. Both physicians and patients judged the lemon balm cream superior to the placebo; it was found, however, that treatment must be started very early in the infection as accelerated healing was most pronounced in the first two days.

Preparations: The dried leaf is available for use as tea. The fresh leaves have a much stronger, more pleasant lemon flavor. Capsules and a cream containing a 1 percent extract are sold in the American market.

Dose: In Germany, 1.5–4.5 g of the herb are steeped in a cup of hot water. Apply cream as directed at early stages of cold sores and genital herpes. (Lemon balm is not approved for treating herpes in the United States.)

Cautions: None noted.

Symptoms

Digestive gas

Herpes sores

Insomnia

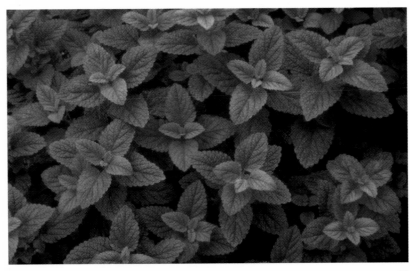

Licorice

Glycyrrhiza glabra

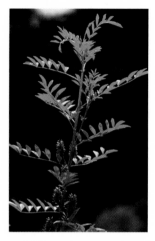

Sources: European licorice is the root of a member of the pea family native to Eurasia. Twenty species of *Glycyrrhiza* are found in Eurasia, North and South America, and Australia. At least six Chinese species are used as Chinese licorice (*gan-cao* or sweet herb), primarily *G. uralensis.* Licorice is cultivated commercially in Europe and Asia.

Traditional Use: What we think of as "licorice" flavor is actually anise; licorice itself tastes very sweet and musty. The Roman naturalist Theophrastus (c. 372–c. 287 B.C.) wrote that the roots were used for asthma, dry cough, and lung disorders. Traditionally, the dried root has also been used for sore throat and laryngitis as well as inflammation of the urinary and intestinal tracts. In China, licorice is first mentioned in *Shen Nong Ben Cao Jing* (first century A.D.). It is used in Chinese prescriptions for coughs, sore throat, asthma, gastric and duodenal ulcers, and as a "mediator" of potentially toxic ingredients.

Current Status: Licorice is considered expectorant, diuretic, anti-inflammatory, and soothing to irritated mucous membranes; it is used in the treatment of inflamed lungs, as well as for gastric and duodenal ulcers. Its cough-suppressant activity resembles that of codeine. It speeds healing of gastric ulcers in part by increasing secretions from the gastric mucosa.

Glycyrrhizin (glycyrrhetic acid) is believed to be the primary active constituent, though other components of licorice contribute to its biological activity. Glycyrrhizin is fifty times as sweet as sugar and is found in licorice at concentrations of 1 to 25 percent. Good-quality licorice should contain at least 4 percent glycyrrhizin.

Licorice is one of the better-studied herbs. Numerous pharmacological and clinical reports confirm its usefulness in treating ulcers and support its reputation as a cough suppressant and expectorant. The German government allows licorice preparations to be used for the supportive treatment of gastric and duodenal ulcers and for congestion of the upper respiratory tract.

Preparations: Licorice is available as whole, sliced, and cut-and-sifted root; in powdered form as capsules and tablets; and as tinctures, extracts, and standardized products. Extracts are used in cough syrups and as flavoring for laxatives.

Dose: In European herbal medicine, products are formulated to deliver an average daily dose of 5–15 g (1–2 tsp) of root (calculated to 200 to 600 mg of glycyrrhizin). Use is limited to four to six weeks, after which side effects may occur.

Cautions: Licorice may cause some individuals to experience water retention and hypertension due to sodium retention and potassium loss. Do not exceed recommended dose. Discontinue use after four to six weeks. Individuals with heart disease, liver disease or hypertension should avoid licorice and it should not be used during pregnancy. If diuretics or heart medications containing digitalis have been prescribed, licorice should be avoided.

Symptoms

Stomach or duodenal ulcers

Actions

Cough suppressant

Expectorant

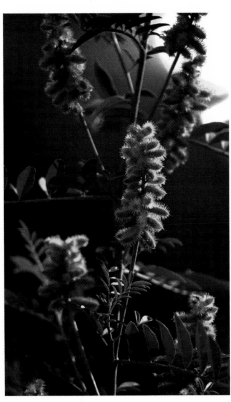

Marshmallow

Althaea officinalis

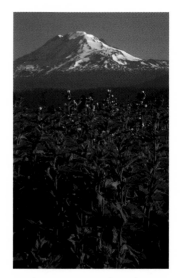

Sources: Marshmallow is the root or leaf of a member of the mallow family that grows in wet soils in much of Europe from England, Denmark, and central Russia south to the Mediterranean region. Escaped from gardens in North America, it grows in salt marshes from Massachusetts to Virginia and in the mountains of the western United States. The root is used to a greater extent than the leaves.

Traditional Use: The genus name *Althaea* comes from the Greek *altho,* "associated with healing". Traditionally, marshmallow root has been poulticed on bruises, muscle aches, sprains, burns, and inflammations. A tea of the leaves has been used to soothe sore throat and as an expectorant in bronchitis and whooping cough. Like many members of the mallow family, its tea is considered soothing to an upset stomach. Both the fresh and dried leaves have been used for similar conditions as the root but are considered somewhat weaker.

Current Status: The leaves and root both contain mucilagin, the substance that makes the tea "slimy", considered the main active ingredient. The leaves contain up to 16 percent mucilagin, while the roots contain 25–30 percent.

Marshmallow preparations are recognized for their ability to soothe and soften irritated tissue, particularly mucous membranes, and to loosen a cough. Marshmallow also mildly stimulates the immune system. The German health authorities allow use of the leaf and root preparations to relieve local irritation and soothe irritated mucous membranes in sore throat accompanied by dry cough. Preparations of the root are also used to relieve local irritations, stimulate the immune system, slow down lung congestion in sore throat with dry cough, and relieve mild inflammation of the mucous membranes of the digestive tract.

Marshmallow

Preparations: Marshmallow root is generally available in the United States. Peeled root is considered of higher quality than root with the outer bark. The leaves are less familiar in America. The whole and cut-and-sifted root and powder are available in teas, capsules, and other formulations. In Europe, marshmallow syrups are available.

Dose: Daily dosage of the dried leaves is up to 5 g (1–2 tsp) divided into two or three doses. That of the root is up to 6 g (1 heaping tsp) divided into two or three daily doses.

Cautions: The mucilagin in marshmallow may absorb and hence reduce the action of drugs taken at the same time. In Germany marshmallow syrups (which are high in sugar) must be labeled as to sugar content so diabetics may be forewarned. Side effects are not reported for marshmallow.

Symptoms

Indigestion
Sore throat

Actions

Expectorant

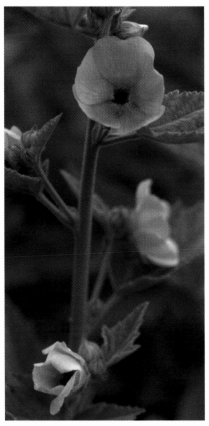

Milk thistle

Silybum marianum

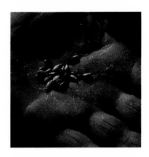

Source: Milk thistle is a member of the aster family found throughout Europe. Introduced by early colonists, it is naturalized in eastern North America and common in California. The seeds are used.

Traditional Use: According to early Greek references, milk thistle seeds have been used to treat liver disorders for over 2,000 years. The Roman writer Pliny the Elder (A.D. 23–79), wrote that the juice of the plant mixed with honey was excellent for "carrying off bile".

Milk thistle is featured in Hildegard of Bingen's *Physica,* the first herbal by a woman, written about 1150 and published in 1533, and other early European herbals mention its use for liver disease. The sixteenth-century English herbalist John Gerard considered it "the best remedy that grows against all melancholy [liver] diseases," and the eighteenth-century German physician Rademacher used the seed for chronic and acute liver diseases. During the next two centuries, its use declined, but by the 1930s, interest in clinical use of milk thistle preparations for liver disease was growing again.

Current Status: More than 300 studies conducted since the late 1960s provide an experimental basis for the effectiveness and safety of silymarin, the main chemical complex of milk thistle seeds, in the treatment of liver disease. Standardized seed preparations have been shown to alter the cell structure of the outer liver membrane which prevents toxic chemicals from entering and stimulates the liver's own capacity to generate new cells. Silymarin also scavenges harmful oxygen radicals in the liver, further protecting it.

German health authorities allow milk thistle preparations to be used in supportive treatment of chronic inflammatory liver disorders such as hepatitis, cirrhosis, and fatty infiltration caused by alcohol or other toxins. In addition to its well-documented curative action, silymarin can help prevent liver damage if it is taken before exposure to toxins.

Preparations: Whole and powdered seeds are available in the American market in capsules, tablets, and tinctures. To ensure predictable effects, however, preparations must be standardized to 70 to 80 percent silymarin (the active constituent).

Dose: The daily dose of standardized products is 420 mg of silymarin divided into three doses. It should be taken for six to eight weeks, after which the dosage can be reduced to 280 mg per day. Traditionally, 12–15 g (2–3 tsp) of the dried powdered seeds are used for tea.

Cautions: There are no serious side effects, contraindications, or drug interactions related to the use of milk thistle preparations. Loose stools may occur during the first few days of use.

Symptoms

Liver disorders

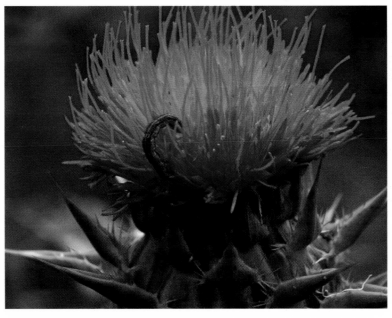

Passionflower

Passiflora incarnata

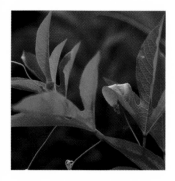

Source: Passionflower is the dried aboveground parts (herb) of a member of the largely tropical American passionflower family, found in fields from Virginia to southern Illinois and southeast Kansas, south to Florida and Texas.

Traditional Use: Passionflower was largely neglected until the mid-nineteenth century. It was introduced into medicine about 1840 by. L. Phares of Mississippi and by 1898 was in use by American physicians. Harvey Wickes Felter and John Uri Lloyd wrote in 1898, "Its force is exerted chiefly upon the nervous system, the remedy finding a wide application in *spasmodic disorders* and as a rest-producing agent. It proves specially useful in the *insomnia* of infants and old people. It gives sleep to those who are laboring under the effects of mental worry or from mental overwork."

Formerly approved as an over-the-counter sedative and sleep aid, it was not recognized as effective by the US Food and Drug Administration in a 1978 review of nighttime sleep aids.

Current Status: Most research on passionflower has been done in animal studies related to its antispasmodic and sedative properties. Extracts of the herb inhibit fungi and bacteria. Studies indicate that the herb (or its extracts) relieves spasms, has a sedative effect, allays anxiety, and lowers blood pressure. In European herbal medicine, passionflower products are used for nervous tension, especially in sleep disturbances or anxiety arising from restlessness. Recent research on passionflower indicates that several chemical components—probably flavonoids—act together to cause these effects. Well-designed clinical research on passionflower alone is notably absent from the literature; a few studies have been done on passionflower in combination with other herbs.

Preparations: The dried herb is generally available and is made into tea, tinctures, fluid extracts, and in Europe, sedative chewing gums. Passionflower is used in European sedatives in combination with

Passionflower

valerian and hawthorn. Passionflower and hawthorn combinations are also used to relieve spasms of the digestive system. For such products, the herb is standardized to contain not less than 0.8 percent total flavonoids to comply with the French, German, and Swiss pharmacopoeias.

Dose: The German health authorities specify a daily dose of 4–8 g (1–2 tsp) of the herb divided into three doses. One-half to 2.5 g (about ½ tsp) of the herb are used to make a cup of tea.

Cautions: Passionflower contains minute amounts of harman alkaloids which can reduce the effects of antidepressants based on monoamine oxidase inhibitors. In Germany, passionflower preparations may contain no more than 0.01 percent of harman alkaloids. Otherwise, no side effects or contraindications are reported for the herb.

Symptoms

Anxiety

Insomnia

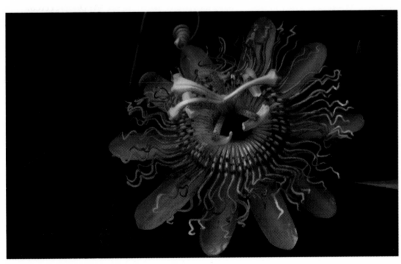

Pau d'arco

Tabebuia impetiginosa (formerly *T. avellanedae*)

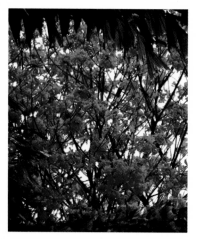

Sources: Pau d'arco is the inner bark or heartwood of a tropical member of the bignonia family found in South America, including Brazil, Peru, and Argentina. Known in the herb trade as lapacho and taheebo, material sold as pau d'arco in the American market may be from other *Tabebuia* species or from tropical trees in the verbena family.

Traditional Use: In the Americas, pau d'arco has a folk reputation as an anticancer, antibacterial, antiviral, and antifungal agent, especially for treating candida infections. Several *Tabebuia* species have long been used by South American indigenous groups as a cancer remedy. In Peru, pau d'arco has been used to treat diabetes and as a blood purifier. It is often used in combination with other herbs. In the late 1960s, popular newspaper and magazine reports in Brazil led to widespread use in South America which prompted scientific research into its purported health benefits.

Current Status: Pau d'arco has been studied for its antitumor, anti-inflammatory, antibacterial, antifungal, and immunostimulant activities. Early results were promising. Immunostimulant action has been examined only in preliminary laboratory studies that did not involve living organisms. Research on anticancer activity was conducted in the late 1960s and early 1970s by the National Cancer Institute. Several chemicals known as quinones have been identified from the bark and heartwood; the primary component, lapachol, was admitted into clinical studies in its pure form but was withdrawn due to lack of substantial benefits and mild toxicity. Advocates of its use argue that the whole bark produces different effects, due to the combined action of dozens of chemicals, that cannot be expected from a single compound. Analyses of commercial products have found that many lack the known active constituents. Pau d'arco is, and is expected to remain, controversial. It is widely used by herbalists outside the

United States to treat cancer; for viral infections such as colds, flu, and herpes; bacterial infections; fungal infections such as candida; inflammations of the nose and throat; and many other conditions.

Preparations: Pau d'arco is available in a wide range of forms including powdered bark, capsules, tablets, tinctures, and extracts.

Dose: The traditional dosage is 15–20 g (2–3 tsp) of the inner bark simmered in a pint of water for 15 minutes, then divided into two or three daily doses. As many as six to nine 300-mg tablets per day have been recommended by herbalists.

Cautions: Reported side effects include nausea and gastrointestinal distress. The toxicity of *T. impetiginosa* is considered relatively low. Other species have produced additional side effects. Pau d'arco should be approached cautiously: its anti-cancer activity is unconfirmed, identification of source species is often questionable, and it is surrounded by enough hype to make anyone skeptical.

Actions

Antibacterial

Antifungal

Antiviral

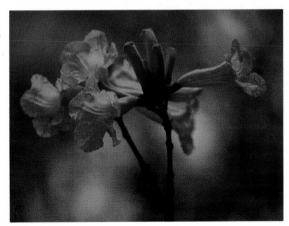

Peppermint

Mentha × piperita

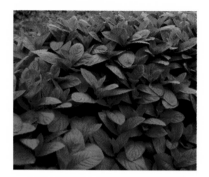

Source: Peppermint is the leaf of a hybrid between spearmint (*M. spicata*) and watermint (*M. aquatica*). Native to Europe, it was first grown commercially in England about 1750. Today peppermint is produced commercially in Indiana, Wisconsin, Oregon, Washington, and Idaho.

Traditional Use: Peppermint is first mentioned in the medical literature of the early 1700s. Samuel Stern described it in 1801 in *The American Herbal:* "It is a stimulant. It restores the functions of the stomach, promotes digestion, stops vomiting, cures the hiccups, flatulent colic, hysterical depressions, and other like complaints." Peppermint leaf tea has been traditionally used for indigestion, nausea, colds, headache, and cramps.

Current Status: Recent research on peppermint has examined its essential oil rather than the leaf. Peppermint oil, which comprises about 0.3 to 0.4 percent of the leaf's weight, has been shown to be antibacterial and antiviral, and it reduces muscle spasms. The primary component is menthol at 30–48 percent of the oil.

A 1979 clinical trial studied use of the oil (in coated capsules so that they dissolve in the intestinal tract rather than the stomach) in eighteen patients with irritable bowel syndrome (colicky abdominal pain and a feeling of distention). One to two capsules were given three times a day, depending upon severity of symptoms, for as long as three weeks. Patients who took the peppermint oil capsules experienced more relief than those who received the placebo. Other researchers confirmed that for peppermint oil to be effective in treating irritable bowel syndrome, the oil had to reach the colon without first being digested in the stomach.

Inhalation of the vigor of peppermint essential oil is thought to help ease congestion from colds and improve breathing by stimulating cold receptors in the respiratory tract. In its 1990 review of over-the-counter drugs, the U. S. Food and Drug Administration dropped the oil from its former status as a nonprescription drug in the United

States, most likely because no data on its safety or effectiveness were submitted by the industry. It is still widely used and approved in Europe.

Preparations: Dried cut-and-sifted leaf, capsules, and tinctures are available in the American market, along with coated capsules of peppermint oil.

Dose: A day's supply of tea is made with 3–6 g (2–4 tsp) of the dried cut-and-sifted leaf and 1.5–3 cups of water. One or two coated peppermint oil capsules, taken three times a day between meals, have been used in clinical studies. Only six to twelve drops a day of the oil is taken, divided into three doses. Follow label instructions; do not exceed recommended doses. For respiratory congestion, put a few drops in a basin of hot water and inhale the vapor with your eyes closed.

Cautions: Coated peppermint oil capsules may sometimes open in the stomach, causing heartburn and relaxation of throat muscles. They should not be used by anyone diagnosed with an absence of hydrochloric acid in gastric juices (achlorhydria). Peppermint oil should not be applied directly to mucous membranes, such as the nostrils, especially of infants and children. The leaf and oil should not be used by anyone with gallbladder or bile duct obstruction, inflammation, or related conditions.

Symptoms

Gastrointestinal spasms
Nausea

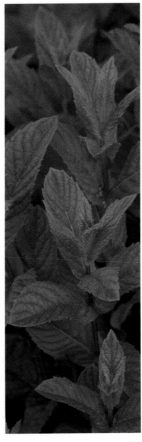

Psyllium

Plantago spp.

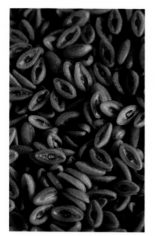

Sources: Psyllium seeds and husks come from three annual species of plantain, a plant group familiar to most as lawn weeds. Blonde psyllium, *P. ovata,* native to the Mediterranean, North Africa, and western Asia, is widely grown in India and Pakistan; black psyllium (*P. psyllium,* and *P. indica,* both known as *P. arenaria*) is native to the Mediterranean region and is commercially grown in Spain and southern France.

Traditional Use: The seeds and fruit husks of psyllium have long been used as bulk laxatives in Europe and the United States.

Current Status: Many consumers may already have psyllium seed products on the shelf as they are a common ingredient in bulk laxatives. The seeds and seed husks contain 10–30 percent mucilage and, when soaked in water, their volume increases greatly, swelling the amount of intestinal matter. This stimulates and lubricates the bowels, encouraging the movement of wastes through the colon. Psyllium seed products are widely prescribed and are also available as nonprescription drugs for the treatment of chronic constipation or to soften the stool to relieve hemorrhoids and related conditions.

In Germany the seeds and husks are also allowed in the supportive treatment of irritable bowel syndrome. Studies have also shown that psyllium produces a modest but significant reduction in cholesterol levels.

Preparations: Dried psyllium seeds and husks are available in the American market, in addition to their presence in many laxative products available at pharmacies.

Dose: The average daily dose is 4–20 g (1 tsp) of the husks or 10–20 g (up to 2 tsp) of the powdered seeds stirred into a large glass of water and taken immediately (before it thickens) 30 minutes to an hour after a meal or after taking other drugs. Follow label instructions on commercial products. If constipation persists, see your doctor.

Cautions: According to German health authorities, psyllium seed and husks are known to produce rare allergic reactions and can be dangerous in cases of intestinal obstruction. Because some psyllium preparations contain sugar, diabetics should use them only under a physician's supervision.

Symptoms

Constipation

Actions

Laxative

Lowers cholesterol

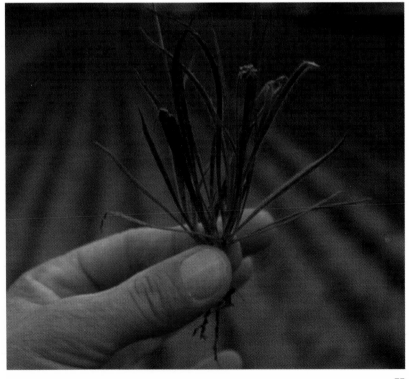

Red clover

Trifolium pratense

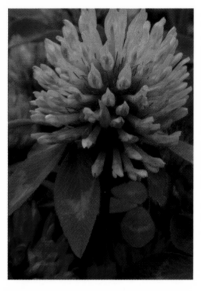

Source: Red clover is the dried flower head of a member of the pea family widely grown as animal fodder and found in temperate climates through the world. It is native to Europe and naturalized throughout the United States.

Traditional Use: Red clover is mentioned as a blood purifier, diuretic, general tonic, and folk cancer remedy in Jethro Kloss's *Back to Eden.* The flower has been used as a folk remedy to relieve spasms associated with asthma and bronchitis and to treat skin sores or ulcerations. It is one of the ingredients of the controversial Hoxsey formula used at alternative cancer clinics in Mexico.

Current Status: Red clover's use as a cancer remedy is not backed by any clinical studies in humans. Pharmacological studies even in animals are few. Red clover does, however, contain an interesting group of compounds called isoflavones, including genistein, diadzen, and biochanin A, among others. James A. Duke has suggested red clover as a good candidate for further examination as a chemopreventive, a dietary substance that may help prevent cancer. Epidemiological studies provide evidence that certain dietary components can have a significant effect on the incidence and location of cancers in humans. For example, some members of the mustard family, especially broccoli, are known to help prevent the development of cancers, an effect attributed to free-radical scavenging properties. The flavonoid genistein (mostly extracted from soybeans) is now available in dietary supplements known as nutraceuticals. A recent preliminary laboratory study found that biochanin A inhibited the activation of cancer in cell cultures. More research on red clover and its isoflavones is clearly warranted.

Red clover

Preparations: Dried red clover tops are generally used in teas, as well as in capsules, tablets, and various combination products.

Dose: Three to 6 g (about 1 tbsp) in tea.

Cautions: No side effects have been reported from using this herb. However, cattle ingesting late season or spoiled red clover hay have developed symptoms such as frothing, diarrhea, dermatitis, and decreased milk production. It is possible that similar effects would occur in persons using fermented or otherwise spoiled red clover.

Actions

Chemopreventive

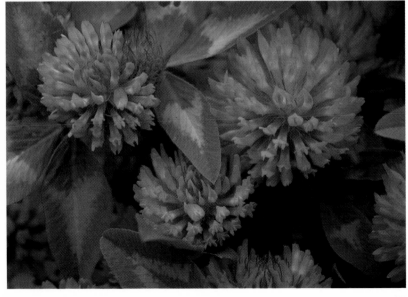

Reishi

Ganoderma lucidum

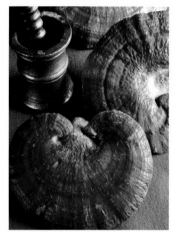

Sources: Known as *reishi* in Japan or *ling-zhi* in China, this herb is the fruiting body of a mushroom. It is produced commercially in China, Japan, and the United States. In Japan it grows in the wild on plum trees, but most of the supply is cultivated. Related species such as artist's conk (*G. applanatum*) occur in North America, but they are not grown commercially nor have their medicinal properties been studied.

Traditional Use: Reishi has been a folk medicine in China for thousands of years. It is mentioned in the first class of herbs in *Shen Nong Ben Cao Jing* for calming, benefiting vital energy (*qi*), and even improving the complexion. Once available only to emperors, this important tonic was considered an "elixir of life". The Chinese name *ling zhi* means "spirit plant"; in traditional Chinese medicine (TCM) it was traditionally used to treat hepatitis, hypertension, arthritis, nervous conditions, insomnia, lung disorders, and as a general tonic to "lighten weight and increase longevity".

Current Status: Reishi's activity is not ascribed to one chemical, but to the collective action of many components, including polysaccharides (which have immunostimulant activity and help to enhance protein synthesis), a heart-toning alkaloid, as well as triterpene acids, which protect the liver, reduce hypertension, and inhibit cholesterol synthesis. Pharmacological studies have confirmed that reishi is antiallergenic, anti-inflammatory, antiviral, antioxidant, immunostimulant, and expectorant, and that it suppresses coughs and increases coronary blood flow. In the past two decades, Asian clinical studies have shown that reishi is effective in treating hepatitis, lowering cholesterol, and relieving bronchitis and asthma. It is also effective in relieving altitude sickness, as a calmative in anxiety and hypertension, and for reducing blood pressure. Reishi preparations are widely used in China and Japan and are increasingly well-known in the West.

Preparations: The dried mushrooms are available in powdered form, capsules, tinctures, tablets, and extracts in the United States. Some products are available in standardized form.

Dose: Three 1 g tablets of the mushroom, taken three times a day.

Cautions: Experimental studies have shown toxicity is very low. Rare side effects include dry throat, nosebleed, and upset stomach after long-term use. Rare skin rashes have also been reported as well as an allergic reaction in one patient who received an injectable form of the drug in China.

Symptoms

Anxiety

Actions

Adaptogen (tonic)

Immunostimulant

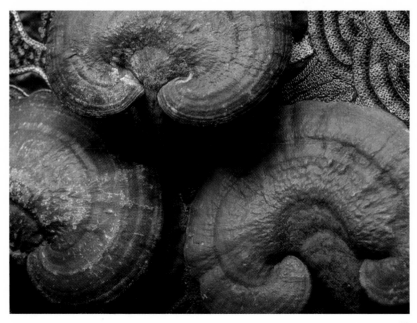

Sarsaparilla

Smilax spp.

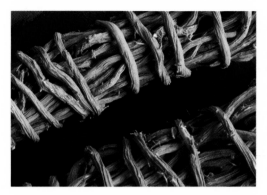

Sources: Sarsaparilla is the root of several South and Central American and Caribbean species of *Smilax*, a genus in the lily family. They include Mexican sarsaparilla (*S. medica*, also known as *S. aristolochiifolia*), Honduran sarsaparilla (*S. regelii*), Ecuadorean sarsaparilla (*S. febrifuga*), Jamaican sarsaparilla (*S. ornata*), and other species. Most of the commercial supply is harvested from the wild.

Traditional Use: Mexican sarsaparilla was exported to Europe before 1530. In sixteenth-century Europe, sarsaparilla was used to treat syphilis and rheumatism. It was official treatment for syphilis in the *U. S. Pharmacopoeia* in 1850. Often an ingredient in patent medicines with extravagant claims in late nineteenth-century America, sarsaparilla products were promoted as blood purifiers, tonics, and diuretics, to induce sweating, and for a myriad of other questionable applications. In recent years sarsaparilla has been touted as a male sexual rejuvenator with claims implying it contains testosterone. It has also been used as an anabolic steroid replacement in natural body-building formulas.

Current Status: Simply put, there is no credible recent research on the actions of sarsaparilla. A few studies in the 1930s and 1940s showed it to be diuretic, anti-inflammatory, and protective of the liver. Benefits were also claimed in cases of eczema and psoriasis. Sarsaparilla does contain plant steroids but nothing close to testosterone, as plant steroids cannot be converted in the body to anabolic steroids or human hormones. The collective scientific evidence, scarce as it is, shows that sarsaparilla is more likely to build profit margins than muscle tissue.

Sarsaparilla extract is approved as a food flavoring ingredient in the United States. In Germany, although it has been traditionally used to treat skin diseases including psoriasis, as well as rheumatism and kidney ailments, products may not carry therapeutic claims because their effectiveness has not been demonstrated. After 500 years of use in the West, sarsaparilla still awaits carefully designed studies.

Preparations: The dried root, powdered root, capsules, tablets, tinctures, and combination products are widely sold in herb markets.

Dose: None noted.

Cautions: According to German health authorities, sarsaparilla preparations have caused stomach irritation and temporary kidney problems. As it is known to increase the absorption of digitalis and hasten the elimination of other medications, thus changing their effective doses, sarsaparilla should not be taken by anyone on prescription medications.

Actions

Flavoring

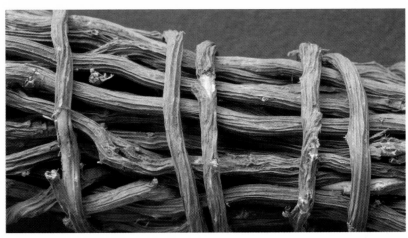

Saw palmetto

Serenoa repens

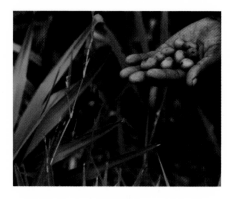

Source: Saw palmetto is the fruit of a small shrub in the palm family native to the southeastern United States from South Carolina to southern Mississippi and throughout Florida. Most of the fruit is wild-harvested in Florida.

Traditional Use: Saw palmetto was introduced into medicine by. J. B. Read, of Savannah, Georgia, in an 1879 issue of the *American Journal of Pharmacy*: "By its peculiar soothing power on the mucous membrane it induces sleep, relieves the most troublesome coughs, promotes expectoration, improves digestion, and increases fat, flesh and strength. Its sedative and diuretic properties are remarkable."

An "original communication" in the July 1892 issue of *The New Idea* stated, "It also exerts a great influence over the organs of reproduction, mammoa, ovarium, prostate, tests [sic], etc. Its action on them is a vitalizer, and is said to be the greatest known, tending to increase their activity and add greatly to their size."

Current Status: Clinical trials with saw palmetto show that it decreases symptoms associated with benign prostatic hyperplasia (BPH), especially reducing the urge to urinate during the night. Fifty percent of men more than fifty years old may develop BPH. Pressure of the enlarged prostate on the bladder may cause many of these men to awaken four or five times a night with an urge to urinate. Components of fat-soluble extracts of the fruit reduce prostate size and inhibit inflammation. A double-blind French clinical trial involving 110 BPH patients, published in 1984, reported that saw palmetto reduced the number of times patients had to urinate at night by more than 45 percent and increased urinary flow rate by more than 50 percent. Painful or difficult urination was significantly reduced in the treatment group as compared to the placebo group. More than 2,000 patients have now been evaluated in clinical trials.

German health authorities allow saw palmetto fruit preparations for difficulty of urination in early stages of BPH.

Preparations: The dried fruit is available in whole or ground form, as well as in capsules, tablets, and tinctures. Benefits are most likely to be achieved with standardized products made with fat-soluble carriers containing high levels of free fatty acids.

Dose: Standardized preparations are taken one or two times a day for a daily dose of 320 mg. The equivalent of 1 to 2 g (½–1 tsp) of the dried fruit is the average daily dose of other preparations.

Cautions: No side effects or contraindications other than rare stomach upset have been reported. The primary condition for which the fruit is used, BPH, can only be diagnosed by a physician, so consult one for proper examination and treatment.

Symptoms

Benign prostatic hyperplasia (BPH)

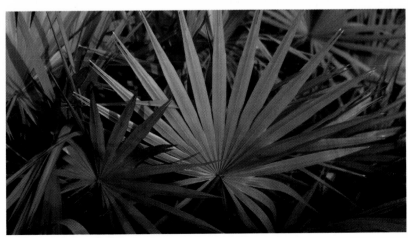

Senna

Cassia acutifolia, C. angustifolia

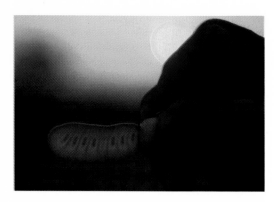

Sources: Senna is the dried leaf or pod of Alexandria senna and Tinnevelley senna. Both species have recently been referred to by botanists as *Senna alexandrina.* They are members of the pea family native to Eurasia, now cultivated commercially in the Middle East and India. Tinnevelley senna is most widely used in the United States.

Traditional Use: Powdered leaf tea has been used for many centuries, both in Eastern and Western traditions, for its laxative qualities.

Current Status: Senna does one thing, and does it well—relieve constipation. Its leaves and pods contain anthranoids which have specific effects in the intestines: chemical by-products of senna metabolism stimulate propulsive contractions and inhibit stationary contractions in the colon, thus speeding elimination of waste and increasing its water and electrolyte content.

Senna leaves contain about half as much of the active compounds as the pods, but they are considered safer to use. Senna is less expensive than cascara sagrada, but it is a stronger laxative with a greater tendency to cause cramping. The leaves, as well as the anthranoids extracted from them, are still official drugs in *U.S. Pharmacopoeia.*

Preparations: Senna is available in a number of product forms including the dried leaf and pods. Because it is a strong laxative, it is best to use commercially prepared non-prescription drug preparations which have more predictable effects.

Dose: Follow instructions on product labels.

Cautions: Senna should not be used for more than a week without a physician's advice. Longer use can cause dependency on laxatives as the bowels may become chronically sluggish. Proper diet and exercise will do much to avoid the need for laxatives. Some individuals may experience discomfort or cramping after using senna products. Prolonged use can lead to fluid and electrolyte imbalances, such as potassium loss, which can reduce the effectiveness of prescribed heart medications. Avoid using senna with licorice root, thiazide diuretics, or steroids because of the potential for potassium loss. Senna should not be used by pregnant or nursing women.

Symptoms

Constipation

Actions

Laxative

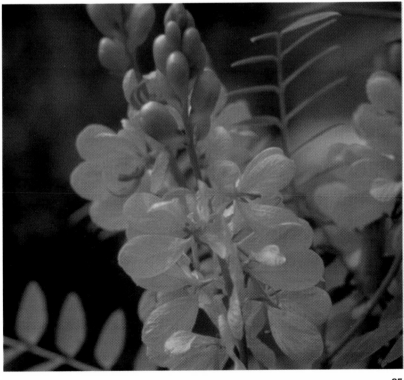

Skullcap

Scutellaria lateriflora

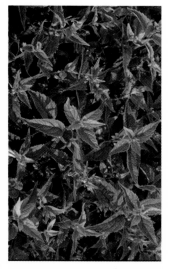

Source: Skullcap is the herb of a member of the mint family from rich woods and moist soils in eastern North America. Another commonly used species is Baikal skullcap, (*S. baicalensis*), the root of which is the Chinese drug *huang-qin.* It is found in sandy fields in northeast China and adjacent Russia and in the mountains of southwest China.

Traditional Use: Also known as maddog skullcap, the American species was historically used to treat rabies. Traditionally it is known as a nerve tonic and sedative for relieving anxiety, neuralgia, and insomnia. Baikal skullcap was first mentioned in the middle class of drugs in *Shen Nong Ben Cao Jing.* In China it is found in prescriptions for fevers, colds, high blood pressure, hypertension, insomnia, headache, intestinal inflammation, vomiting of blood, and other conditions.

Current Status: Almost all recent research has been done on the Chinese *S. baicalensis.* Few studies have been done on American skullcap, but one of its compounds, scutellarin, has been shown to have mild sedative and antispasmodic properties. Baikal skullcap, the subject of numerous Chinese studies, inhibits bacteria and viruses, is diuretic, and lowers fevers and blood pressure; in China, it is used to treat hepatitis. One flavonoid found in the root, baicalin, has similar properties. Clinical studies in China show that a tincture of Baikal skullcap reduces high blood pressure.

American skullcap is a good candidate for further research.

Preparations: Skullcap is available in dried form as teas, capsules, tablets, and tinctures. Care should be taken to buy skullcap from a reliable source to ensure the identity of the plant material.

Dose: In Chinese tradition, 3–9 g of the root are simmered in tea.

Cautions: Recently several herbs, including European products containing germander (*Teucrium chamaedrys*), have been linked to liver damage. The North American native germander (*T. canadensis*), also known as wood sage or wild basil, has traditionally been used to induce menstruation, urination, and sweating. It is widely seen as an adulterant in commercial supplies of skullcap (*S. lateriflora*). Reports of liver toxicity related to skullcap may actually involve the adulterant, which is traded as "pink skullcap". Two cases of "skullcap" poisoning, including one fatality, were reported from the Riks Hospital in Oslo, Norway, in 1991. It is unclear whether the offending herb was *S. lateriflora* or a species of *Teucrium*.

Actions

Sedative, mild

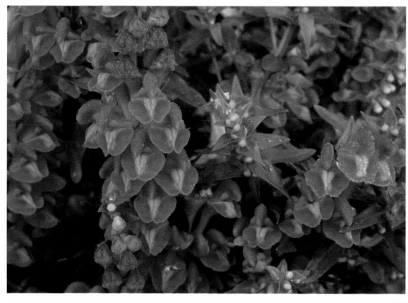

Slippery elm

Ulmus rubra

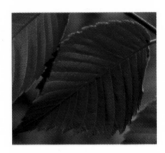

Sources: Slippery elm is the inner bark of a tree in the elm family, formerly known as *U. fulva,* native from Maine through the St. Lawrence valley, west to the Dakotas, south to Texas, and east to Florida. The bark is harvested from wild trees; the rough outer bark is removed and the inner bark retained.

Traditional Use: Slippery elm was one of the most useful medicinal plants of the American wilderness. Native Americans from the Missouri River Valley used a tea of the fresh inner bark to make a soothing laxative. Among the Creek, a poultice of the bark was a toothache remedy. The Osage and other groups applied bark poultices to extract thorns and gunshot balls. Surgeons during the American Revolution used bark poultices as their primary treatment for gunshot wounds, and a soldier, separated from his company, survived for ten days in the wilderness on slippery elm and sassafras barks. During the War of 1812, when food was scarce, British soldiers fed their horses on slippery elm bark. Nineteenth-century physicians recommended slippery elm broth as a wholesome and nutritious food for infants and invalids, and the tea has long been the herbal treatment of choice for acute stomach ulcers and colitis. Adopted as an official drug for the first *U. S. Pharmacopoeia* in 1820, slippery elm was listed until 1936.

Current Status: Slippery elm is a good example of an herb that works well for a particular purpose which has not been disputed. The inner bark contains high amounts of mucilage, made up of starch, polysaccharides, and low levels of tannins. When water is added to the powdered bark, the "slippery" brew is soothing to irritated mucous membranes of the intestinal tract, as well as the throat. It is still approved by the Food and Drug Administration as a nonprescription product for demulcent use.

Preparations: Cut-and-sifted and powdered bark are available. Only a handful of herb milling plants produce slippery elm powder, as it is highly combustible. Lozenges containing slippery elm are sold in the American market.

Dose: One-half to 2 g (about ½ tsp) of the powdered bark added to a cup of hot water for tea and taken two or three times daily.

Cautions: No side effects or special cautions are noted.

Symptoms

Convalescence

Gastrointestinal irritation

Sore throat

Actions

Nutritive

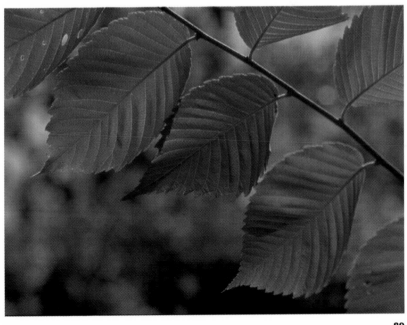

St.-John's-wort

Hypericum perforatum

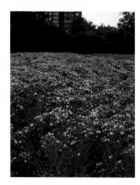

Source: St.-John's-wort is the dried herb or flowering top of a member of the St.-John's-wort family, native to Europe and naturalized in Asia, Africa, North America, South America, and Australia. In 1793 the first recorded specimen in the United States was collected in Pennsylvania. Commercial supplies come from plants cultivated and wild-harvested in Chile, the United States, and Europe.

Traditional Use: St.-John's-wort has interested herbalists since the first-century Greek physicians Galen and Dioscorides recommended it as a diuretic, wound-healing herb, and treatment for menstrual disorders. During the Middle Ages, remarkable, even mystical properties were attributed to it—St.-John's-wort was thought to be best if harvested on St. John's Day (June 24). In nineteenth-century America, it was used by physicians for wound healing, especially for lacerations involving damaged nerves, and as a diuretic, astringent, and mild sedative.

Current Status: Eighteen double-blind clinical trials in humans indicate that standardized St.-John's-wort preparations are safe and effective in the treatment of depression and have far fewer side effects than conventional drugs. A recent clinical trial confirmed the results of previously reported studies. In a randomized placebo-controlled double-blind study of 105 outpatients diagnosed with mild to moderate depression or temporary depressive moods, patients were given the equivalent of 300 mg of St.-John's-wort extract (standardized to a hypericin content of 0.9 mg) or a placebo daily for four weeks. In the treatment group, 67 percent improved, but only 28 percent of the placebo group responded. Patients who took the extract felt significant improvement in depressive mood indicators such as feelings of sadness, hopelessness, helplessness, and uselessness, as well as fear and difficult or disturbed sleep. No significant side effects were observed. Researchers concluded that St.-John's-wort extract, compared with synthetic antidepressants, produced side effects of minor significance and can be recommended for the treatment of mild and moderate

St.-John's-wort

depression. Externally, St.-John's-wort oil is used for the treatment of wounds, abrasions, and first-degree burns.

Preparations: The dried herb and flowering tops may be made into tea or soaked in olive oil (imparting a red pigment, hypericin, to the oil) and used for external applications. Products standardized to contain 0.2 to 0.3 percent hypericin are now available. Capsules, tablets, tinctures, extracts and other products are also found in the American market.

Dose: A daily dose of 2–4 g ($^1/_2$–1 tsp) of the dried herb (containing 0.2–1.0 mg hypericin) is used in tea. Extracts standardized to 0.3 percent hypericin are taken in doses of 300 mg three times a day to deliver 1 mg of hypericin daily.

Cautions: Hypericin from the flowers may cause light-skinned animals that consume the plant to break out in hives or blisters upon exposure to sunlight, a reaction called photodermatitis. If you have fair skin, be aware of this potential problem, especially if you are likely to be exposed to bright sunlight after taking the herb. Clinical studies on St.-John's-wort extract's antidepressant activity have not reported this side effect, but in studies using pure hypericin, photodermatitis did occur in humans.

Symptoms

Cuts and abrasions

Actions

Antidepressant

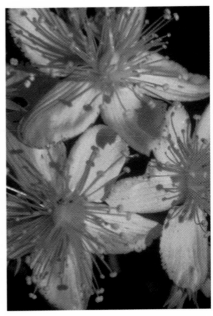

Stinging nettle

Urtica dioica

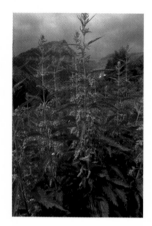

Sources: Stinging nettle is a perennial member of the nettle family, native to both Europe and the United States. The root and leaf are used.

Traditional Use: In folk medicine, the dried herb and fresh plant juice have been used as diuretics, astringents and blood builders, and to treat anemia (due to their high iron content). The powdered leaves or fresh leaf juice have been applied to cuts to stop bleeding or taken in tea to reduce excessive menstrual flow, as well as to treat nosebleeds and hemorrhoids. Nettle tea has been used to stimulate blood circulation and as a spring tonic for chronic skin ailments. France's official bulletin on herbal medicines notes that it is traditionally used for the treatment of mild acne and eczema. It is also a folk treatment for arthritis.

Current Status: Recent studies suggest that the leaf tea aids coagulation and formation of hemoglobin in red blood cells. A freeze-dried nettle leaf product has shown slight activity in the treatment of allergies. Several studies indicate that the leaf extract depresses the central nervous system and inhibits bacteria and adrenaline. Stinging nettle's diuretic activity has been the subject of a number of German studies. Animals fed stinging nettle showed increased excretion of chlorides and urea. The juice has a distinctly diuretic effect in patients with heart disorders or chronic venous insufficiency. The herb's high potassium content and flavonoids may contribute to its diuretic action. In Germany, the herb is used for supportive treatment of rheumatic complaints and kidney infections.

Stinging nettle root is attracting new research interest. German health authorities allow root preparations of stinging nettle to be used for symptomatic relief of urinary difficulties associated with early stages of benign prostatic hyperplasia (BPH), although they don't decrease enlargement of the prostate. The root preparation increases urinary output and decreases the urge to urinate at night. Studies suggest that the root extract may inhibit interaction between a growth factor and its receptor in the prostate. Patients must consult a physician regularly for proper monitoring of the treatment.

Preparations: The dried leaf, used as tea, or capsules, tablets, and tinctures are available. Dried root products, often combined with saw palmetto, have begun to appear on the American market.

Dose: In Germany an average daily dose of 8–10 g (1–2 tbsp) of the dried herb is used for supportive treatment of rheumatic complaints, inflammation of the lower urinary tract, and for treatment of renal gravel. For root preparations, an average daily dose of 4–6 g (about 1 tsp) can be made into a cup of tea and divided into two or three doses.

Cautions: Fresh nettle leaves sting! The burning sensation usually lasts for about an hour, but may persist for up to twelve hours in some individuals. Histamine, acetylcholine, 5-hydroxytryptamine, small amounts of formic acid, leukotrienes, and other unknown compounds act together to produce the sting. No side effects or contraindications are reported for nettle products. The primary condition for which the roots are used, BPH, can be diagnosed only by a physician.

Symptoms

Benign prostatic hyperplasia (BPH)

Actions

Diuretic

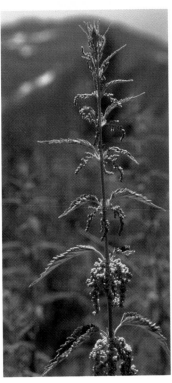

Tea tree

Melaleuca alternifolia

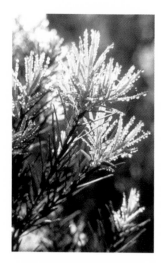

Sources: Tea tree is a small tree in the myrtle family that grows in wet ground on the northern coast of New South Wales and southern Queensland, Australia. The essential oil is produced commercially on plantations in New South Wales.

Traditional Use: Interest in tea tree oil emerged in the 1920s when Australian researchers found it had up to thirteen times greater antiseptic activity than carbolic acid, then a well-known germicide. In 1930, *The Medicinal Journal of Australia* revealed that the oil, when applied to carbuncles and pus-filled infections, dissolved pus and inhibited bacterial growth without damaging surrounding tissues. Further studies established the oil as a disinfectant in soaps, a topical treatment for parasitic skin diseases, and a deodorant for wounds. A couple of drops in a glass of water were recommended as a gargle for sore throat at early stages of inflammation. Its confirmed antiseptic activity, gentleness to oral mucosa, and apparent lack of toxicity endeared it to Australian dentists. Physicians used the oil to treat throat infections, dirty wounds, candida, and fungal infections including ringworm and athlete's foot.

Current Status: Tea tree oil is now one of Australia's more popular herbal exports. A 1990 clinical trial involving 124 patients provides evidence of its effectiveness in the treatment of facial acne. A 5 percent solution of tea tree oil in a water-based gel was less effective (because of slower onset of action) than 5 percent benzoyl peroxide in a water-based lotion, but was better tolerated by facial skin with less scaling, dryness, itching, and irritation than with the benzoyl peroxide preparation.

A recent multicenter, randomized, double-blind clinical study of 117 patients found that 100 percent tea tree oil applied topically to fungus-infected toenails was as effective as a standard treatment of 1 percent clotrimazole solution. Another recent study found that tea tree oil had strong activity against antibiotic-resistant bacteria strains.

Preparations: The essential oil is generally available, as are vaginal suppositories for candida. In the mid-1980s, an Australian quality standard for tea tree oil was established, calling for a component known as terpinen-4-ol to constitute 30 percent or more of the oil, with less than 15 percent cineole, a compound considered to reduce the oil's quality. The standard has some latitude, with higher quality oils containing 40–47 percent terpinen-4-ol, and only 2.5 percent cineole. Oils high in terpinen-4-ol and low in cineole are considered best for predictable results.

Dose: Apply topically as directed on product labels.

Cautions: None noted, though as with all essential oils, some individuals may experience contact dermatitis. Internally, all essential oils are potentially toxic. Use only as directed.

Symptoms

Acne

Candida

Actions

Antibacterial

Antifungal

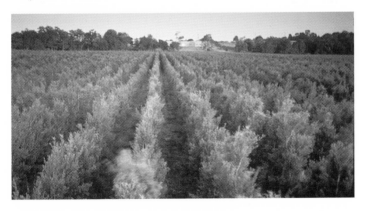

Valerian

Valeriana officinalis

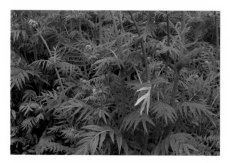

Sources: Valerian is the root of a perennial member of the valerian family found in eastern, southeastern, and east-central Europe, to south Sweden and the southern Alps. It escaped from cultivation in the northeastern United States and is commercially grown in Europe, the United States, and elsewhere.

Traditional Use: Valerian, not a major medicinal plant of the ancient classical authors, was best known to them as a diuretic and treatment for menstrual difficulties. The Greek physician Galen used it for epilepsy in children and adults. An Italian nobleman, Fabio Colonna, born in 1567, suffered from epilepsy and found Galen's reference. He took valerian himself and claimed it completely restored his health. His words stimulated interest in the plant as a sedative. Use of valerian to relieve spasms and as a sleep aid evolved in the seventeenth and eighteenth centuries. Valerian was an official remedy in the *U. S. Pharmacopoeia* from 1820 to 1936.

Current Status: Valerian is widely used in Europe as a mild nerve sedative and sleep aid for insomnia, excitability, and exhaustion. Experimental studies have shown that it depresses the central nervous system and relieves muscle spasms. Its sedative action is attributed to a number of chemical fractions, with no single compound emerging as the active principle.

In the 1980s Swiss researchers studied the effects of valerian water extracts on sleep patterns. Sleep quality was assessed by the patients and by laboratory measures. The time taken to fall asleep was reduced, especially in older patients and insomniacs. Dream recall and nocturnal movement were apparently not affected. No hangover effect, a common complaint among users of synthetic sedatives, was reported the following morning. German health authorities allow use of valerian in sedative and sleep-inducing preparations for states of excitation and for difficulty in falling asleep due to nervousness.

Valerian

Preparations: Dried valerian root is available in whole, cut-and-sifted, and powdered form for teas, capsules, tablets, tinctures, extracts, and other preparations. Some products are standardized to contain at least 0.5 percent essential oils.

Dose: The standard daily dose is 2–3 g (about ½ tsp) of the root divided into two or three doses each day. Products standardized to 0.5 percent essential oil may be taken at a dose of 300 to 400 mg per day. As a sleep aid valerian is taken one hour before bedtime.

Cautions: Some individuals may experience temporary stomach upset. Compounds called valepotriates have been shown to destroy and cause mutations in animal cells. Despite these findings, valerian is generally considered safe. Although official texts do not caution against using valerian during pregnancy, avoid it to be on the safe side.

Symptoms

Anxiety

Insomnia

Actions

Sedative, mild

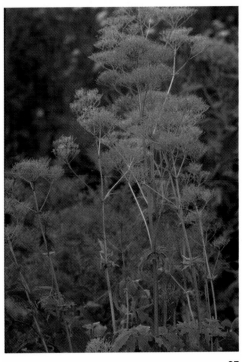

Vitex

Vitex agnus-castus

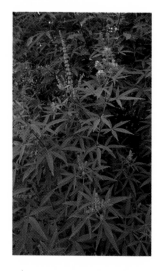

Sources: Vitex, or chaste tree, is the fruit of a shrub in the verbena family native to west Asia and southwestern Europe. It was introduced throughout Europe at an early date and is naturalized in much of the southeastern United States. The fruits are grown commercially in Europe.

Traditional Use: Vitex has been used for menstrual difficulties for at least 2,500 years. Hippocrates (460–377 B.C.) wrote, "If blood flows from the womb, let the woman drink dark wine in which the leaves of the vitex have been steeped." Its use for gynecological conditions is also noted in the works of Pliny (A.D. 23–79): "The trees furnish medicines that promote urine and menstruation." In the late 1800s American physicians used a tincture of the fresh berries to increase milk secretion and treat menstrual disorders.

Current Status: During the past forty years, research has focused on the use of vitex for premenstrual syndrome (PMS) and menstrual difficulties. The biological activity cannot be attributed to a single chemical ingredient, though flavonoids are major components.

Between 5 and 30 percent of women may be affected by PMS. A 1992 survey of German gynecologists evaluated the effect of a vitex preparation on 1,542 women diagnosed with PMS. Both physicians and patients assessed effectiveness, with 90 percent reporting relief of symptoms after treatment averaging 25.3 days.

In one clinical drug-monitoring study on the effectiveness and safety of long-term treatment with a vitex fruit tincture, 1,571 women with menstrual disorders and PMS were followed for a period of seven days to six years (average 147.6 days). In 90 percent of patients, the treatment eliminated or alleviated symptoms of PMS.

German health authorities allow vitex preparations for disorders of the menstrual cycle, pressure and swelling in the breasts, and PMS. In Germany, vitex preparations are frequently used in the safe and effective treatment of PMS, heavy or too frequent periods, acyclic bleeding, infertility, suppressed menses, and other conditions. Vitex is an excellent example of an herbal medicine which serves as a low-priced tool in European gynecological practice, rather than as an "alternative" to conventional treatment.

Preparations: Most European clinical studies have been done on a proprietary extract (tincture) and capsules called Agnolyt. In the United States the dried fruit is available in whole or pulverized form, capsules, tinctures, tablets, and other preparations.

Dose: Preparations are formulated so an average daily dose is equivalent to 30–40 mg of the berries divided into two or three doses or 40 drops of a standardized tincture or one capsule each day. Results can be expected in four to eighteen months.

Cautions: Do not use vitex if you are pregnant or receiving hormone replacement therapy. Rare side effects include early menstruation following delivery (resulting from activation of the pituitary), as well as rare cases of itching, rashes, and gastrointestinal symptoms. In clinical trials, side effects have been reported in fewer than 2 percent of patients.

Symptoms

Menopausal difficulties

Menstrual difficulties

PMS

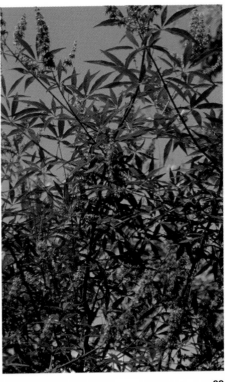

Willow

Salix spp.

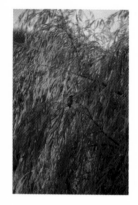

Sources: Willow is the inner bark of several species of Salix, trees in the willow family including white willow (*S. alba*). Four other European species recognized as sources are crack willow (*S. fragilis*), purple willow (*S. purpurea*), violet willow (*S. daphnoides*), and bay willow (*S. pentandra*). All except bay willow are naturalized in North America.

Traditional Use: For more than 2,000 years, people of the Northern Hemisphere used willow bark as a wash for external ulcers and internally to reduce fevers and relieve aches, pains, rheumatism, arthritis, and headaches. Native Americans used it: black willow root bark was used by the Houma as a blood thinner; the Creek used the root tea to relieve inflammation in rheumatism and to reduce fever. In American folk traditions, the bark was used as a blood thinner (like aspirin) and to treat fever. The tea was also given for dyspepsia. In 1763, a Dr. Stone of London first recommended willow bark to the medical profession for the treatment of fevers.

Current Status: In the 1890s the Bayer Company was looking for a substitute for wintergreen and black birch oil, then used to relieve pain, because they were simply too toxic. Their researchers studied experiments from 1853 in which salicylic acid was first synthesized from carbolic acid. They rediscovered a derivative of the acids developed in the 1853 studies—"acetylsalicylic acid", commonly known today as aspirin. No other drug is as well-known for its analgesic, fever-reducing or anti-inflammatory qualities. Willow bark has been considered a "natural aspirin".

Willow bark contains compounds called phenolic glycoside esters. Intestinal micro-organisms transform these compounds to saligenin, which is oxidized in the liver and blood, producing salicylic acid. It has pain-relieving effects like aspirin, but with fewer side effects. Pain is reduced by inhibition of prostaglandin synthesis in sensory nerves. The question then becomes whether you can take enough willow bark to achieve this effect? According to Varro Tyler, probably not.

Preparations: The dried bark is available in whole form or pulverized for teas, capsules, tablets, and other products. In Europe, willow products standardized to salicin are available. Bark should contain at least 1 percent salicin.

Dose: A standard dose is 1–2 g ($\frac{1}{4}$–$\frac{1}{2}$ tsp) of the powdered bark (corresponding to 20–40 mg of salicin). Taken three times a day, it could deliver as much as 120 mg of salicin. Varro Tyler calculates that, due to the low salicin content of most commercial willow bark, it would take between three pints and five quarts of willow bark tea to provide a single dose of salicin equivalent to a dose of aspirin. Therefore, it would be difficult to achieve a similar therapeutic effect.

Cautions: Willow bark is high in tannins, which can damage the liver. Because willow bark produces salicin, it is suggested to be contraindicated in the same instances as aspirin for stomach ulcers and, in children, for high fevers. However, salicin does not metabolize the same as aspirin, so the contraindications may not apply.

Symptoms

Fever

Aches and pains

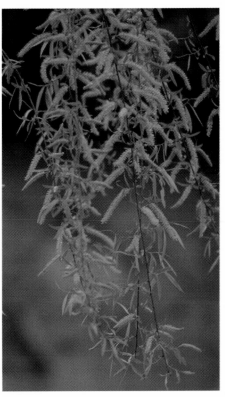

Therapeutic Cross-Reference List

The following list is intended as a quick reference guide to symptoms and conditions for which the listed herbs have clinically proven effects. Before using an unfamiliar herb, you should be careful to read the full profile, especially the cautions.

aches and pains	Willow
acne	Tea tree
angina pectoris	Hawthorn
anxiety	Hops, Kava-kava, Passionflower, Reishi, Valerian
appetite, lack of	Hops
asthma, mild	Ephedra
atherosclerosis	Bilberry
benign prostatic hyperplasia (BPH)	Saw palmetto, Stinging nettle
burns, first degree	Aloe, Calendula
candida	Tea tree
colds	Astragalus, Echinacea
congestive heart failure, early stages	Hawthorn
constipation	Cascara sagrada, Psyllium, Senna
convalescence	Ginseng, Slippery elm
cuts and abrasions	Aloe, Gotu kola, St.-John's-wort
diarrhea	Bilberry
essential fatty acids deficiency	Evening primrose oil
fatigue	Ginseng
fever	Willow
flu	Astragalus, Echinacea
gas, digestive	Lemon balm
gastrointestinal irritation or inflammation	Goldenseal, Slippery elm
gastrointestinal spasms	Peppermint
hemorrhoids	Bilberry

herpes sores	Lemon balm
indigestion	Chamomile, Ginger, Marshmallow
infections, minor	Astragalus, Echinacea
insomnia	Chamomile, Hops, Kava-kava, Lemon balm, Passionflower, Valerian
liver disorders	Milk thistle
memory loss, age-related	Ginkgo
menopausal difficulties	Black cohosh, Dong-quai, Vitex
menstrual difficulties	Black cohosh, Dong-quai, Vitex
migraine headaches	Feverfew
motion sickness	Ginger
mouth and throat inflammation	Bilberry, Calendula
mucous membrane inflammation	Goldenseal
nasal congestion	Ephedra
nausea	Chamomile, Ginger, Peppermint
PMS	Black cohosh, Dong-quai, Evening primrose oil, Vitex
sore throat	Calendula, Marshmallow, Slippery elm
stress	Gotu kola, Kava-kava
tendency to bruising	Bilberry
tinnitus	Ginkgo
ulcers, stomach or duodenal	Licorice
urinary tract infections, mild	Bearberry, Cranberry
varicose veins	Bilberry

Bibliography

Herb References

Alfalfa

Bradley, B. A. "Uses of Alfalfa." In *Observation with Medicago Sativa.* Cincinnati, Ohio: Lloyd Brothers, 1915.

Olin, B. R., ed. "Alfalfa." *Lawrence Review of Natural Products* (March 1991).

Aloe

Grindlay, D., and T. Reynolds. "The *Aloe vera* Phenomenon: A Review of the Properties and Modern Uses of the Leaf Parenchyma Gel." *Journal of Ethnopharmacology* 16 (1986): 117–151.

Heggers, J. P., R. P. Pelley, and M. C. Robson. "Beneficial Effects of *Aloe* in Wound Healing." *Phytotherapy Research* 7 (1993): S48–S52.

Koo, M. W. L. *"Aloe vera*: Antiulcer and Antidiabetic Effects." *Phytotherapy Research* 8 (1994): 461–464.

Leung. A. *"Aloe vera* Update: A New Form Questions Integrity of Old." *Drug & Cosmetic Industry* (September 1985): 42–46.

Saito, H. "Purification of Active Substances of *Aloe arborescens* Miller and their Biological and Pharmacological Activity." *Phytotherapy Research* 7 (1993): S14–S19.

Astragalus

Chu, D. A., et al. "Immunotherapy with Chinese Medicinal Herbs II. Reversal of Cyclphophamide-induced Immune Suppression by Administration of Fractionated *Astragalus membranaceus in vivo.*" *Journal of Clinical and Laboratory Immunology* 25 (1988): 125–129.

Sun, Y., et al. "Immune Restoration and/or Augmentation of Local Graft Versus Host Reaction by Traditional Chinese Medicine Herbs." *Cancer* 52(1) (1983): 70–73.

Bearberry

ESCOP. *Proposals for European Monographs,* vol. 3. Bevrijdingslaan, Netherlands: European Scientific Cooperative for Phytotherapy, 1992.

Bilberry

Bettini, V., et. al. "Effects of *Vaccinium myrtillus anthocyanoside* on Vascular Smooth Muscle." *Fitoterapia* 55(5) (1984): 265–272.

Cunio, L. *"Vaccinium myrtillus."* *Australian Journal of Medical Herbalism* 5(4) (1993): 81–85.

Lietti, A., and G. Forni. "Studies of *Vaccinium myrtillus anthocyanosides* I. Vasoprotective and Anti-inflammatory Activity." *Arnzeimittel Forschung-Drug Research* 26 (1976): 829–832.

Black cohosh

Düker, E.M., et al. "Effects of Extracts from *Cimicifuga racemosa* on Gonadotropin Release in Menopausal Women and Ovariectomized Rats." *Planta Medica* 57 (1991): 420–424.

Lehmann-Willenbrock, E., and H. H. Riedel. *Zentralblatt für Gynäkologie* 110(10) (1988): 611–618.

Calendula

Della Loggia, R., et al. "The Role of Triterpenoids in the Topical Anti-Inflammatory Activity of *Calendula officinalis* Flowers." *Planta Medica* 60 (1994): 516–520.

ESCOP. *Proposals for European Monographs,* vol. 3. Bevrijdingslaan, Netherlands: European Scientific Cooperative for Phytotherapy, 1992.

Olin, B. R., ed. "Calendula." *Lawrence Review of Natural Products* (January 1995).

Cascara sagrada

Tyler, V. E., L. R. Brady, and J. E. Robbers. *Pharmacognosy,* 9th ed. Philadelphia: Lea & Febiger, 1988.

Cat's-claw

Aquino, R., et al. "Plant Metabolites, New Compounds, and Anti-Inflammatory Activity of *Uncaria tomentosa*." *Journal of Natural Products* 54(2) (1991): 453–459.

Duke, J. "Una de Gato." *The Business of Herbs* (May/June 1994).

Jones, K. *Cat's-claw—Healing Vine of Peru.* Seattle: Sylvan Press, 1995.

Rizzi, R., et al. "Mutagenic and Antimutagenic activities of *Uncaria tomentosa* and Its Extracts." *Journal of Ethnopharmacology* 38 (1993): 63–67.

Stuppner, H., et al. "A Differential Sensitivity of Oxindole Alkaloids to Normal and Leukemic Cell Lines." *Planta Medica* 59 (1993) Supplement: 583.

Wagner, H., et al. "Die Alkaloide von *Uncaria tomentosa* und ihre Phagozytose-steigernde Wirkung." *Planta Medica* 51 (1985): 419–423.

Cayenne

Palevitch, D., and L. Craker. "Nutritional and Medical Importance of Red Pepper (*Capsicum* spp.)." *Journal of Herbs, Spices & Medicinal Plants* 3(2) (1995): 55–83.

Chamomile

ESCOP. *Proposals for European Monographs,* vol. 1. Bevrijdingslaan, Netherlands: European Scientific Cooperative for Phytotherapy, 1990.

Foster, S. "Chamomile." Botanical Series, no. 307. Austin, Texas: American Botanical Council, 1991.

Salamon, I. "Chamomile in Slovakia." *The Herb, Spice and Medicinal Plant Digest* 10(1) (1992): 1–4.

Cranberry

Avorn, J., et al. "Reduction of Bacteriuria and Pyuria After Ingestion of Cranberry Juice." *Journal of the American Medical Association* 271(10) (1994): 751–754.

Ofek, I., et al. "Anti-Escherichia coli Adhesion Activity of Cranberry and Blueberry Juices." *New England Journal of Medicine* 324 (1991): 1599.

Zafari, D., et al. "Inhibitory Activity of Cranberry Juice on Adherence of Type 1 and Type P Fimbriated Escherichia coli to Eucaryotic Cells." *Antimicrobial Agents and Chemotherapy* 33 (1989): 92–98.

Dandelion

ESCOP. *Proposals for European Monographs,* vol. 3. Bevrijdingslaan, Netherlands: European Scientific Cooperative for Phytotherapy, 1992.

Hobbs, C. *"Taraxacum Officinale:* A Monograph and Literature Review." In *Eclectic Dispensatory of Botanical Therapeutics,* vol. 1. Portland, Oregon: Eclectic Medical Publications 1989: 6-156–6-205.

Dong-quai

Belford-Cortney, R. "Comparison of Chinese and Western Uses of *Angelica sinensis.*" *Australian Journal of Medical Herbalism* 5(4) (1993): 87–91.

Chang, H. M., and P. P. H. But, eds. *Pharmacology and Applications of Chinese Materia Medica,* vol. 1. Singapore: World Scientific, 1986.

Echinacea

Bauer R., and Wagner, H. "Echinacea Species as Potential Immunostimulatory Drugs." In *Economic and Medicinal Plant Research,* vol. 5. Orlando, Florida: Academic Press, 1991: 253–320.

Bräunig, B., et al. *"Echinacea purpurea* radix for Strengthening the Immune Response in Flu-like Infections." *Zeitschrift für Phytotherapie* 13 (1992): 7–13.

Foster, S. *Echinacea: Nature's Immune Enhancer.* Rochester, Vermont: Healing Arts Press, 1991.

Melchart, D., et al., "Immunomodulation with Echinacea—A Systematic Review of Controlled Clinical Studies." *Phytomedicine* 1 (1994): 245–254.

Eleuthero

Farnsworth, N. R., et al. "Siberian Ginseng (*Eleutherococcus senticosus*): Current Status as an Adaptogen." In *Economic and Medicinal Plant Research,* vol. 1. Orlando, Florida: Academic Press, 1985: 155–215

Foster, S. "Siberian Ginseng, *Eleutherococcus senticosus.*" *Botanical Series,* no. 302. Austin, Texas: American Botanical Council, 1991.

Ephedra

Chen, K. K. "Half a Century of Ephedrine." *American Journal of Chinese Medicine* 2(4) (1974): 359–365.

Kalix, P. "The Pharmacology of Psychoactive Alkaloids from Ephedra and Catha." *Journal of Ethnopharmacology* 32 (1991): 201–208.

Evening primrose

Briggs, C. J. "Evening Primrose: *La Belle de Nuit,* The King's Cureall." *Canadian Pharmaceutical Journal* (May 1986): 249–254.

Horrobin, D. F. "Gamma Linolenic Acid." *Reviews in Contemporary Pharmacology* 1 (1990): 1–45.

Khoo, S. K., et al. "Evening Primrose Oil and Treatment of Premenstrual Syndrome." *Medical Journal of Australia* 153 (1990): 189–192.

Feverfew

Awang, D. V. C. "Feverfew." *Canadian Pharmaceutical Journal* 122(5) (1989): 266–70.

Awang, D. V., et al. "Parthenolide Content of Feverfew (*Tanacetum parthenium*) Assessed by HPLC and ¹H-NMR Spectroscopy." *Journal of*

Natural Products 54(6) (1991): 1516–21.

Foster, S. "Feverfew—*Tanacetum parthenium.*" *Botanical Series,* no. 310. Austin, Texas: American Botanical Council, 1991.

Johnson, E. S., et al. "Efficacy of Feverfew as a Prophylactic Treatment of Migraine." *British Medical Journal* 291 (1985): 569–573.

Murphy, J., et al. "Randomized, Double-Blind, Placebo-Controlled Trial of Feverfew in Migraine Prevention." *The Lancet* (July 23, 1988): 189–192.

Fo-ti

Grech, J. N., et. al. "Novel CA^{2+}-AtPase Inhibitors from the Dried Root of *Polygonum multiflorum.*" *Journal of Natural Products* 57(12) (1994): 1682–1687.

Hong, C. Y., et al. "*Astragalus membranaceus* and *Polygonum multiflorum* Protect Rat Heart Mitochondria Against Lipid Peroxidation." *American Journal of Chinese Medicine* 22(1) (1994): 63–70.

Horikawa, K., et al. "Moderate Inhibition of Mutagenicity and Carcinogenicity of Benzo[a]purene, 1,6-dinitropyrene, and 3,9-dinitroflouranthene by Chinese Medicinal Herbs." *Mutagensis* 9(6) (1994): 523–26.

Garlic

Foster, S. "Garlic—*Allium sativum.*" *Botanical Series,* no. 311. Austin, Texas: American Botanical Council, 1991.

Koch, H. P., and L. D. Lawson, eds. *Garlic—The Science and Therapeutic Application of* Allium sativum L. *and Related Species,* 2nd ed. Baltimore: Williams & Wilkins, 1995.

Reuter, H. D. "*Allium sativum* and *Allium ursinum:* part 2, Pharmacology and Medicinal Application." *Phytomedicine* 2(1) (1995): 73–91.

Ginger

Awang, D. V. C. "Ginger." *Canadian Pharmaceutical Journal* (July 1992): 309–311.

Bone, M. E., et al. "Ginger root —A New Antiemetic. The effect of ginger root on postoperative nausea and vomiting after major gynecological surgery." *Anesthesia* 45(8) (1990): 669.

Grontved, A., et al. "Ginger Root Against Seasickness." *Acta Otolaryngol (Stockh)* 105 (1988): 45–49.

Holtmann, S., et al. "The anti-motion sickness mechanism of ginger." *Acta Otolaryngol (Stockh)* (1989): 108, 168.

Mowrey, D. B., and D. E. Clayson. "Motion Sickness, Ginger and Pyschophysics." *Lancet 20* (1982): 655–667.

Wood, C. D., et al. "Comparison of Efficacy of Ginger with Various Antimotion Sickness Drugs." *Clinical Research Practices and Drug Regulatory Affairs* 6(2)(1988): 129–136.

Yamahara, et. al. "Gastrointestinal Motility Enhancing Effect of Ginger and its Active Constituents." *Chemical and Pharmaceutical Bulletin* 38(2) (1990): 430–431.

Ginkgo

DeFeudis, F. V. *Ginkgo biloba* Extract (EGb 761): *Pharmacological Activities and Clinical Applications.* Amsterdam: Elsevier, 1991.

Foster, S. *"Ginkgo biloba." Botanical Series,* no. 304. Austin, Texas: American Botanical Council, 1991.

Fünfgeld, E. W., ed. *Rökan (Ginkgo biloba), Recent Results in Pharmacology, and Clinic.* Berlin: Springer-Verlag, 1988.

Kleijnen, J., and P. Knipschild. "Ginkgo biloba for cerebral insufficiency." *British Journal of Clinical Pharmacology* 34 (1992): 352–358.

Sohn, M., and R. Sikora. "Ginkgo biloba extract in the therapy of erectile dysfunction." *Journal of Sex Education and Therapy* 17 (1991): 53–61.

Ginseng

Foster, S. "Asian Ginseng, *Panax ginseng.*" *Botanical Series,* no. 303. Austin, Texas: American Botanical Council, 1991.

———. American Ginseng, *Panax quinquefolius. Botanical Series,* no. 308. Austin, Texas: American Botanical Council, 1991.

Hu, S. Y. "The Genus *Panax* (Ginseng) in Chinese Medicine." *Economic Botany* 30 (1976): 11–28.

———. "A Contribution to Our Knowledge of Ginseng." *American Journal of Chinese Medicine* 5 (1977): 1–23.

Ng, T. B., and H. W. Yeung. "Scientific Basis of the Therapeutic Effects of Ginseng." In *Folk Medicine, The Art and the Science* Washington, D.C.: American Chemical Society, 1986: 139–151.

Shibata, S., O. Tanaka, J. Shoji, and H. Saito. "Chemistry and Pharmacology of *Panax.*" In *Economic and Medicinal Plant Research,* vol. 1. Orlando, Florida: Academic Press, 1985: 218–284.

Goldenseal

Combie, J., T. E. Nugent, and T. Tobin. "Inability of Goldenseal to Interfere with the Detection of Morphine in Urine." *Equine Veterinary Science* (January/February 1982): 16–21.

Foster, S. "Goldenseal—Masking of Drug Tests from Fiction to Fallacy: An Historical Anomaly." *HerbalGram* 21 (1989): 7, 35.

———. "Goldenseal *Hydrastis canadensis." Botanical Series,* no. 309. Austin, Texas: American Botanical Council, 1991.

Genest, K., and D. W. Hughes. "Natural Products in Canadian Pharmaceuticals IV *Hydrastis Canadensis.*" *Canadian Journal of Pharmaceutical Science* 4 (1969): 41–45.

Gotu kola

Diwan, P. V., et al. "Anti-Anxiety Profile of Manduk Parni (*Centella Asiatica*) in Animals." *Fitoterapia* 62 (1991): 3, 253–257.

Kartnig, T. "Clinical applications of *Centella asiatica* (L.) Urb. In *Herbs, Spices, and Medicinal Plants—Recent Advances in Botany, Horticulture and Pharmacology,* vol. 3. Phoenix: Oryx Press, 1988: 145–193.

Morisset, R., et al. "Evaluations of the Healing Activity of Hydrocotyle Tincture in the Treatment of Wounds." *Phytotherapy Research* 1(3) (1987): 117–121.

Nalini, N., et al. "Effect of *Centella asiatica* Fresh Leaf Aqueous Extract on Learning and Memory and Biogenic Amine Turnover in Albino Rats." *Fitoterapia* 63(3) (1992): 232–237

Hawthorn

Hamon, N. W. "Herbal medicine: Hawthorns (Genus *Crataegus*)." *Canadian Pharmaceutical Journal* 121 (1988): 708–709, 724.

Hobbs, C., and S. Foster. "Hawthorn—A Literature Review." *HerbalGram* 22 (1989): 18–33.

Lloyd, J. U. "A Treatise on *Crataegus.*" *Drug Treatise* no. 29. Cincinnati: Lloyd Brothers Pharmacists, 1921.

Hops

ESCOP. *Proposals for European Monographs,* vol. 1. Bevrijdingslaan, Netherlands: European Scientific Cooperative for Phytotherapy, 1992.

Kava-kava

Lebot, V., et al. *Kava—The Pacific Drug.* New Haven, Connecticut: Yale University Press, 1992.

Lemon balm

Wöbling, R. H., and K. Leonhardt. "Local therapy of herpes simplex with dried extract from *Melissa officinalis.*" *Phytomedicine* 1(1) (1994): 25–31.

Licorice

Hayashi, H., et al. "Distribution Pattern of Saponins in Different Organs of *Glycyrrhiza glabra.*" *Planta Medica* 59 (1993): 351–353.

Kimura, Y., et al. "Effects of Flavonoids from Licorice Roots (*Glycyrrhiza inflata* Bat.) on Arachidonic Acid Metabolism and Aggregation in Human Platelets." *Phytotherapy Research* 7 (1993): 341–347.

Nielsen, I., and R. S. Pederson. "Life-threatening hypokalaemia caused by licorice ingestion." *Lancet* 2 (1984): 1305.

Marshmallow

Ninov, S., et al. "Constituents of *Althaea officinalis* var. 'Russalka' Roots." *Fitoterapia* 63 (1992): 474.

Tomoda, M., et al. "Hypoglycemic Activity of Twenty Plant Mucilages and Three Modified Products." *PlantaMedica* 53 (1987): 8–12.

Milk thistle

Foster, S. "Milk Thistle *Silybum marianum.*" *Botanical Series* no. 305. Austin, Texas: American Botanical Council, 1991.

Hikino, H., and Y. Kiso. "Natural Products for Liver Disease" In *Economic and Medicinal Plant Research,* vol. 2. New York: Academic Press, 1988: 39–72.

Leng-Peschlow, E., and A. Strenge-Hesse. "The Milk Thistle (*Silybum marianum*) and *Silymarin* in Liver Therapy." *Phytotherapie* 12(5) (1991): 162–174.

Salmi, H. A., and S. Sarna. "Effect of *Silymarin* on Chemical, Functional, and Morphological Alterations of the Liver: A Double-blind Controlled Study." *Scandanavian Journal of Gastroenterololology* 17 (1982): 517–521.

Passionflower

ESCOP. *Proposals for European Monographs,* vol. 2. The Netherlands: European Scientific Cooperative for Phytotherapy, 1992.

Foster, S. "The Passionflowers." *The Herb Companion* (August/September 1991): 18–23.

Olin, B. R., ed. "Passion Flower." *The Lawrence Review of Natural Products.* May 1989.

Speroni, E., and A. Minghetti. "Neuropharmacological Activity of Extracts from *Passiflora incarnata*." *Planta Medica* 54 (1988): 488–491.

Pau d'arco

Awang, D. V. C., et al. "Naphthoquionone Constituents of Commercial Lapacho/Pau D'Arco/Taheebo Products." *Journal of Herbs, Spices, and Medicinal Plants* 2(4) (1994): 27–43.

Block, J. B., et al. "Early Clinical Studies with Lapachol." *Cancer Chemotherapy Reports,* part 2, 4(4) (1974): 27–28.

Jones, K. *Pau d'Arco.* Rochester, Vermont: Healing Arts Press, 1995.

Oswald, E. H. "Lapacho." *British Journal of Phytotherapy* 3(3) (1993/94): 112–117.

Peppermint

ESCOP. *Proposals for European Monographs,* vol. 3. Bevrijdingslaan, Nether-lands: European Scientific Cooperative for Phytotherapy, 1992.

Foster, S. "Peppermint—*Mentha piperita.*" *Botanical Series* no. 306. Austin, Texas: American Botanical Council, 1991.

Rees, W. D. W., B. K. Evans, and J. Rhodes. "Treating Irritable Bowel Syndrome with Peppermint Oil." *British Medical Journal.* (October 6, 1979): 835–836.

Somerville, K. W., C. R. Richmond, and G. D. Bell. "Delayed Release of Peppermint Oil Capsules (Colpermin) for the Spastic Colon Syndrome: A Pharmacokinetic Study." *British Journal of Clinical Pharmacology* 18 (1984): 638–640.

Stearn, S. *The American Herbal.* Walpole, New Hampshire: Thomas and Thomas, 1801: 227–228.

Psyllium

ESCOP. *Proposals for European Monographs,* vol. 2. Bevrijdingslaan, Netherlands: ESCOP Secretariat, 1992.

Sprecher, D. L., et al. "Efficacy of psyllium in reducing serum cholesterol levels in hypercholesterolemic patients on high- or low-fat diets." *Annals of Internal Medicine* 119(7) (1993): 545–554.

Red clover

Cassady, J. M., et al. "Use of Mammalian Cell Culture Benzo(a)pyrene Metabolism Assay for the Detection of Potential Anticarcinogens from Natural Products: Inhibition of Metabolism by Biochanin A, an Isoflavone from *Trifolium pratense* L." *Cancer Research* 48 (1988): 6257–6261.

Duke, J. A. "Red Clover." *Business of Herbs* (September/October 1990): 8–9.

Yanagihara, K., et al. "Antiproliferative effects of Isoflavones on Human Cell Cancer Lines Established from the Gastrointestinal Tract." *Cancer Research* 53 (1993): 5815–5821.

Reishi

Hobbs, C. *Medicinal Mushrooms: An Exploration of Tradition, Healing and Culture.* Santa Cruz, California: Botanica Press, 1995.

Sarsaparilla

Hobbs, C. 1988. "Sarsaparilla—A Literature Review." *HerbalGram* 17 (1988): 1, 10–15.

Saw palmetto

Champault, G., et al. "The Medical Treatment of Prostatic Adenoma— A Controlled Study: PA-109 versus Placebo in 110 Patients." *Annals of Urology* 6 (1984): 407–410.

Hale, E. M. *Saw Palmetto.* Philadelphia: Boericke & Tafel, 1898.

Senna

Leng-Preschlow, E., ed. "Senna and Its Rational Use." *Pharmacology* 44(S1) (1992): 1–52.

Skullcap

Anon. "Scullcap Substitution." *HerbalGram* (Fall 1985): 3.

Huxtable, R. J. "The Myth of Beneficent Nature: The Risks of Herbal Preparations." *Annals of Internal Medicine* 117(2) (1992): 165–166.

Leander, S., and L. Skogstrøm. "Natural Medicine Can Cause Liver Damage." *Aflenposten,* November 6, 1991.

Slippery Elm

Foster, S. "Slippery Elm." *Business of Herbs* (March/April 1991).

Tyler, V. and S. Foster. "Herbs and Phytomedicinal Products." In *Handbook of Nonprescription Drugs,* 11th ed. Washington, D.C.: American Pharmaceutical Association, 1996: 701–702.

St.-John's-wort

Awang, D. V. C. "St. John's Wort." *Canadian Pharmaceutical Journal* 124 (1991): 33–35.

Harrer, G., and H. Sommer. "Treatment of Mild/Moderate Depressions with *Hypericum.*" *Phytomedicine* 1(1) (1994): 3–8.

Suzuki, O., et al. "Inhibition of Monoamine Oxidase by Hypericin." *Planta Medica* 50 (1984): 272–274.

Stinging nettle

Belaiche, P., and O. Lievoux. "Clinical Studies on the Palliative Treatment of Prostatic Adenoma with Extract of *Urtica* Root." *Phytotherapy Research* 5 (1991): 267–269.

Gansser, D., and G. Spiteller. "Aromatase inhibitors form *Urtica dioica* Roots." *Planta Medica* 61 (1995): 138–140.

Hirano, T., et al. "Effects of Stinging Nettle Root Extracts and Their Steroidal Components on the Na^+, K^+-ATPase of the Benign Prostatic Hyperplasia." *Planta Medica* 60 (1994): 30–33.

Patten G. "Urtica." *Australian Journal of Medical Herbalism* 5(1) (1993): 5–13.

Tea-tree

Bassett, I. B., et al. "A Comparative Study of Tea Tree Oil Versus Benzoylperoxide in the Treatment of Acne." *Medical Journal of Australia* 153(8) (1990): 455–458.

Buck, D. S., et al. "Comparison of Two Topical Preparations for the Treatment of Onychomycosis: *Melaleuca alternifolia* (Tea Tree) Oil and Clotrimazole." *The Journal of Family Practice* 38(6) (1994): 601–605.

Carson, C. F., et al. "Susceptibility of Methicillin-Resistant *Staphylococcus aureus* to the Essential Oil of

Melaleuca alternifolia." *Journal of Antimicrobial Chemotherapy* 38(6) (1995): 421–424.

Foster, S. "Tea Tree and Its Relatives." *The Herb Companion* (February/March 1994): 48–52.

Valerian

Chauffard, F., et al. "Detection of Mild Sedative Effects: Valerian and Sleep in Man." *Experimentia* 37 (1982): 622

ESCOP. *Proposals for European Monographs,* vol. 1. Brussels: European Scientific Cooperative for Phytotherapy, 1990.

Foster, S. "Valerian—*Valeriana officinalis.*" *Botanical Series,* no. 312. Austin, Texas: American Botanical Council, 1991.

Hobbs, C. "Valerian *Valeriana officinalis:* A Literature Review." *HerbalGram* 21 (Fall 1989): 19–34.

Houghton, P. J. "The Biological Activity of Valerian and Related Plants." *Journal of Ethnopharmacology* 22 (1988): 121–142.

Leathwood, P. D., F. Chauffard, E. Heck, and R. Munoz-Box. "Aqueous Extract of Valerian Root (*Valeriana officinalis*) Improves Sleep Quality in Man. Reduces Sleep Latency to Fall Asleep in Man." *Pharmacology Biochemistry & Behavior* 17 (1982): 65–71.

Vitex

Böhnert, K.-J., and G. Hahn. "Phytotherapy in Gynecology and Obstetrics—*Vitex agnus-castus* (Chaste Tree)." *Acta Medica Emperica* 9 (1990): 494–502.

Brown, D. *"Vitex agnus-castus* Clinical Monograph." *Quarterly Review of Natural Medicine* (Summer 1994): 111–121.

Coeugniet, E., E. Elek, and R. Kühnast. "Premenstrual Syndrome (PMS) and

its Treatment." *Ärztezeitschrift für Naturheilverf* 27(9) (1986): 619–622.

Dittmar, F. W., et al. "Premenstrual Syndrome (PMS): Treatment with a Phytopharmaceutical." *TW. Gynäkol* 5(1) (1992): 60–68.

Feldmann, H. U., M. Albrecht, M. Lamertz, and K.-J. Böhnert. "The Treatment of Corpus Luteum Insufficiency and Premenstrual Syndrome: Experience in a Multicentre Study under Practice Conditions." *Hygne* 11(12) (1990): 421.

Willow

Julkunen-Tiitto, R., and B. Meier. "The Enzymatic Decomposition of Salicin and Its Derivatives Obtained from Salicaceae Species." *Journal of Natural Products* 55(9) (1992): 1204–1212.

Tyler, V., and S. Foster. *Herbs and Phytomedicines in Handbook of Nonprescription Drugs,* 11th ed. Washington, D.C.: The American Pharmaceutical Association, 1996.

General References

Blumenthal, M., ed., S. Klein, trans. *German Commission E Therapeutic Monographs on Medicinals Herbs for Human Use.* Austin, Texas: American Botanical Council, 1996.

Bradly, P. R., ed. *British Herbal Compendium,* vol. 1. Dorset, England: British Herbal Medicine Association, 1992.

Brown, D. *Herbal Prescriptions for Better Health.* Rocklin, Calif.: Prima Publishing, 1996.

Christopher, J. *School of Natural Healing.* Springville, Utah: Christopher Publications, 1996.

Duke, James A. *Handbook of Medicinal Herbs.* Boca Raton, Florida: CRC Press, Inc., 1986.

Felter, H. W. and J. U. Lloyd. *King's American Dispensatory,* 2 vols. Portland, Ore.: Eclectic Medical Publications, reprinted 1983.

Foster, S. *Herbal Renaissance.* Layton, Utah: Gibbs Smith Publisher, 1993.

Foster, S. and J. A. Duke. *A Field Guide To Medicinal Plants: Eastern and Central North America.* Boston: Houghton Mifflin Co., 1990.

Foster, S. and C. X. Yue. *Herbal Emissaries: Bringing Chinese Herbs to the West.* Rochester, Vt: Healing Arts Press, 1992.

Grieve, M. *A Modern Herbal,* 2 vols. New York: Hafner, 1967.

Kloss, J. *Back to Eden.* Coalmont, Tenn.: Longview Publishing House, 1939.

Leung, A. Y. and S. Foster. *Encyclopedia of Common Natural Ingredients Used in Food, Drugs, and Cosmetics,* 2nd. ed. New York: John Wiley & Sons, 1996.

Thompson, S. *New guide to Health of Botanic Family Physician.* Boston, Mass.: J. Q. Adams, 1835.

Tyler, V. E. *The Honest Herbal,* 3rd ed. Binghamtom, New York: Pharmaceutical Products Press, 1993.

Tyler, V. and S. Foster. "Herbs and Phytomedicinal Products." In *Handbook of Nonprescrition Drugs,* 11th ed. Washington, D.C.: American Pharmaceutical Association, 1996: 695–713.

———. *Herbs of Choice—The Therapeutic Use of Phytomedicinals.* Binghamtom, New York: Pharmaceutical Products Press, 1994.

Weiss, R.F. *Herbal Medicine* (translated from the German by A.R. Meuss). Beaconsfield, England: Beaconsfield Publishers Ltd., 1988.

Wren, R. C., revised by E. M. Williamson and F. J. Evans, *Potter's New Cyclopedia of Botanical Drugs and Preparations,* 8th ed. Essex: C. W. Daniel Co., 1988.

Glossary

acne vulgaris   Chronic skin disease, common during adolescence, characterized by eruptions of pimples

acyclic bleeding   Menstrual bleeding with abnormal timing

adaptogen   Human health enhancer [see Betsy note on edited fax]

adrenaline   Hormone secreted by the adrenal glands that raises blood pressure and stimulates the heart

alkaline   Higher than 7 on the pH scale, a standard of acidity or alkalinity of solutions; 7 is neutral, below 7 is acidic.

anabolic steroid   Usually synthetic hormones that increase metabolism, sometimes used illicitly by athletes to increase muscle mass.

analgesic   Substance that relieves pain.

anaphylactic shock   Extreme sensitivity to foreign substances such as wasp venom, causing serious, life-threatening symptoms.

anemia   Deficiency of red blood cells, hemoglobin, or total blood volume.

angina pectoris   Transient chest pain caused by inadequate oxygenation of heart muscle.

anti-inflammatory   Reducing inflammation.

antioxidant   Substance that prevents oxidation by free radicals, which causes cell damage that may lead to chronic diseases such as cancer.

antiseptic   Substance that inhibits the growth of microorganisms.

arrhythmia   Irregular heartbeat.

arteriosclerosis   Hardening of the arteries.

astringent   Serving to draw together soft tissue.

atherosclerosis   Type of arteriosclerosis characterized by fatty deposits in the arteries.

atherosclerotic plaque   Fatty deposit in an artery.

atopic eczema   Dermatitis caused by allergy.

Ayurveda   The ancient traditional medicine system of India, encom-passing spiritual, philosophical, and physical principles. Hundreds of herbs are used in Ayurvedic medicine.

benign prostatic hyperplasia (BPH)   Nonmalignant prostate enlargement, often leading to constriction of the urethra, commonly experienced by men over 50.

bronchodilator   Substance that relaxes bronchial muscle's, expanding bronchial air passages.

candida   A yeastlike fungus in the genus *Candida* that occurs normally in the mouth, vagina, and intestines but can proliferate due to disruption of normal flora. *C. albicans* causes thrush. [per Betsy's editing, this last sentence no longer applies without elucidation.]

capillary fragility   Condition in which smallest blood vessels are easily broken.

carminative   Expelling digestive gas.

chemopreventive   Agent that prevents development of cancer.

cholesterol   White, soapy, fatty constituent of animal cells and fluids associated with arteriosclerosis.

coagulation Transformation of a liquid into a mass or clot.

collagenasis Disorder [Disease? see Betsy note] of connective fibers in bone, cartilage, and tissue.

colon The largest section of the large intestine.

congestive heart failure Disorder characterized by inadequate blood output, diminished circulation, edema.

contact dermatitis Skin inflammation caused by touching a noxious plant or other substance.

cough suppressant Substance that reduces the severity of a cough.

crossover trial Clinical trial in which subjects receive both the test substance and a placebo during the course of the study.

cystitis Inflammation of the urinary bladder.

cytotoxic Destructive to cells.

decoction Preparation made by simmering plant parts in water.

degradation Decomposition of a compound or reduction of its complexity.

demulcent Agent that soothes irritated inner core membranes.

dermabrasion Surgical removal of skin blemishes and scars by friction.

dermatitis Inflammation of the skin.

diaphoretic Agent that increases perspiration.

digitalis Dried powdered leaf of foxglove (Digitalis purpurea), a strong heart stimulant and diuretic.

diuretic Agent that promotes urination.

double-blind Relating to a study in which neither researcher nor subject knows whether the subject receives the test substance or a placebo.

dysentery Infection of the lower intestinal tract resulting in severe diarrhea.

dyspepsia Mild indigestion, often accompanied by gas.

eczema Noncontagious inflammation of the skin characterized by redness, itching, and weeping blisters.

edema Accumulation of watery fluid in connective tissue; dropsy

electrolyte Substance in solution which carries an electrical charge, for example, ionized sodium, calcium, or potassium salts in the body or blood plasma.

enteritis Inflammation of the intestines.

epidemiological Pertaining to the study of the incidence, distribution, and control of disease in a population.

epilepsy Chronic disorder of the central nervous system characterized by convulsions.

essential fatty acids Compounds that are not manufactured by the body but, like vitamins, minerals, and essential amino acids, are necessary for good health. Safflower, corn, cottonseed, soybean, and canola oils, as well as flaxseed and leafy green vegetables, are good dietary sources.

estrogen Hormone secreted by the ovaries.

expectorant Agent that promotes expulsion of mucous from the respiratory tract.

flatulence   Excessive gas in the digestive tract.

free fatty acids   Class of organic acids in an unattached, uncombined, or available form.

free radical   Reactive atom or group of atoms having at least one unpaired electron that causes cell damage that may lead to cancer. (See also antioxidant.)

gastric mucosa   Mucous membrane of the stomach. [see Betsy note]

glaucoma   Disease of the eye characterized by increased pressure in the eyeball that can cause gradual loss of vision.

gonorrhea   Infectious inflammation of the genital mucous membrane; sexually transmitted disease.

granulation   Formation of small projections on a wound indicating that healing has begun.

herpes simplex   Virus infection marked by watery blisters on the lips or genitals.

high blood pressure   hypertension

high-density lipoproteins   Relatively small-molecular-weight fats in the blood correlated with reduced risk of atherosclerosis; "good cholesterol".

hyperacidity   Abnormal degree of acidity in the stomach.

hypertension   Abnormally high arterial blood pressure.

hypotensive   Characterized by or causing low blood pressure.

impotence   In the male, inability to copulate.

infusion   Product obtained by steeping herbs in hot water.

ingestion   Introduction of food or drink into the digestive tract.

irritant laxative   Substance that relieves constipation by irritating the colon.

laceration   A torn and ragged wound.

laxative   Substance used to relieve constipation.

lesion   Wound or injury.

leukosis   Abnormal proliferation of white blood cells.

luteinizing hormone   A hormone secretion of the pituitary gland.

metabolism   Utilization of nutrients by the body to produce energy for vital processes and activities.

migraine   Recurrent incapacitating headache, often accompanied by nausea.

monoamine oxidase inhibitor   Drug used to combat depression.

multiple sclerosis   Slow progressive disease of the central nervous system associated with paralysis and muscle tremor.

mutagenic   Capable of changing the hereditary material in a gene or chromosome.

neurotransmitter   Substance that transmits nerve impulses between nerve cells.

nutraceutical   Plant-derived compound essential to nutrition, with additional health benefits. [Betsy questions last phrase]

peristalsis   Waves of involuntary contraction by smooth muscles of the digestive tract that propel the contents onward.

pituitary gland Endocrine organ attached to the brain whose secretions affect most body functions including growth and the menstrual cycle.

placebo Inert or innocuous substance.

placebo controlled Referring to a clinical study that compares a test substance controlled with an inert or innocuous substance to determine effectiveness or safety.

platelet aggregation Collation of blood platelets into a mass.

premenstrual syndrome (PMS) Group of symptoms experienced by some women before menstruation that may include irritability, headache, edema, depression, etc.

prostaglandin Any of various fatty acids that perform a variety of hormone-like actions in animals (such as controlling blood pressure).

[**pruritus** Betsy advises we delete this entry since all it means is itch.]

psoriasis Chronic skin disease characterized by red patches covered with white scales.

qi In Chinese medicine, vital energy; life force.

renal gravel Small masses of mineral salts in the kidneys.

restorative Returning health to normal.

retinopathy Noninflammatory disorder of the retina of the eye.

scurvy Disease caused by vitamin C deficiency.

sedative Tranquilizer; relaxant.

[**sleep aid** Betsy says drop this since everybody know's what it means]

steroids Any of numerous compounds containing a 17-carbon 4-ring system. Examples include cholesterol, glycosides, and various hormones.

systemic lupus erythematosus (SLE) Inflammatory connective-tissue disease that occurs chiefly in women.

systemic vasodilation T cell Expansion of the blood vessels. [see long note] Specialized cell in the blood that controls cellular immunity.

testosterone Hormone that induces and maintains male secondary sex characters.

thiazide Any of a group of drugs used as oral diuretics, especially in the control of high blood pressure.

tinea Any of several fungal diseases of the skin, especially ringworm.

tinnitus Ringing in the ears.

tonic Substance that increases body tone. [see note]

topical Applied externally, usually to the skin.

U.S. Pharmacopoeia A compendium of drugs recognized by the U. S. medical community and government as safe and effective.

vascular Relating to or containing blood vessels.

venous insufficiency Disorder in which superficial veins are dilated, slowing down blood flow. [see note]

Index